Clinical Perspectives in
Nursing Research

RELEVANCE, SUFFERING, RECOVERY

Papers presented at the fourteenth annual
Stewart Conference on Research in Nursing
sponsored by
the Department of Nursing Education and
the Nursing Education Alumni Association
Teachers College, Columbia University
March 1976

Clinical
Perspectives in
Nursing Research

RELEVANCE, SUFFERING, RECOVERY

M. Janice Nelson, EDITOR

TEACHERS COLLEGE PRESS
Teachers College, Columbia University
New York & London

Published by Teachers College Press
            1234 Amsterdam Avenue
            New York, N. Y. 10027

Manufactured in the United States of America

Library of Congress Cataloging in Publication Data

Stewart Nursing Research Conference, 14th, Columbia University, 1976.
     Clinical perspectives in nursing research.

     Includes bibliographies.
     1. Nursing—Congresses.   2. Nursing—Study and teaching—Congresses.
3.   Nursing—Psychological aspects—Congresses.   4.   Nursing—Research—Congresses
     I. Nelson, M. Janice, 1928-   II. Columbia University. Teachers College. Dept. of
Nursing Education.   III.   Columbia University. Nursing Education Alumni Association.
IV.   Title. [DNLM: 1.   Students, Nursing—Congresses. 2.   Education, Nursing—Congresses.   3.   Patients—Congresses.   4.   Pain—Congresses. 5.   Acute
disease—Congresses.   6.   Convalescence—Congresses.   W3   ST313   14th
 1976c / WY18   S845   1976c] RT3.S74 1976   610.73   78-18242

ISBN 0-8077-2549-8

Preface

THE RESEARCH reports contained in this monograph were selected from those presented at the fourteenth annual Stewart Conference on Research in Nursing held at Teachers College, Columbia University, in March, 1976.

As research endeavors in nursing gain momentum, it is important to discern different dimensions of the multifaceted phenomena that present themselves to nurses as they go about the daily business of delivering health care services. In keeping with this notion, this publication introduces three dimensions that are critical both to nursing education and to nursing practice.

These reports are of particular interest and importance because they represent a healthy combination of the scientific on the one hand, while attending to individual perspectives on the other. In other words, while employing various modes of sound scientific inquiry, these authors also focused on personal perception, individual inference, and experience of nursing students, professional nurses, and clients. The Allerman and Britten study, for example, is concerned with students' perceptions of the clinical laboratory. Results revealed that nursing students in their sample did not always regard their clinical experiences as meaningful in translating nursing theory into nursing practice. The Oberst study sought to determine how professional nurses view patients' suffering. This author concluded that nursing's knowledge base for understanding and identifying suffering among patients is scant and, in some respects, inaccurate. Finally, the Kolditz and Naughton study revealed that patients' perceptions of their recovery from acute illness have broad implications for the nursing process in general and for effective discharge planning in particular.

Although editorial constraints do not allow for inclusion of all the discussion following these presentations, critiques of the studies are included in order to allow the reader some insight into the proceedings of the sessions.

Acknowledgments for their efforts contributing to the success of the conference are extended to the principal investigators and to those who critiqued their studies. They are also extended to the faculty of the Department of Nursing Education and to the officers of the Nursing Education Alumni Association, whose joint efforts made the conference possible. Thanks are also extended to those students in the Department of Nursing Education who gave so unstintingly of their time and of themselves to see that every last detail was accounted for. Finally, acknowledgments are extended to the 1976 Stewart Conference Planning Committee: M. Leah Gorman, Dorothy Ozimek, Mary T. Ramshorn, and Dorothy Nayer. Special thanks are extended to Miss Yaye Togasaki, Executive Secretary of the Nursing Education Alumni Association, whose gracious assistance and generosity contributed much toward making the conference the success it most assuredly was.

M. JANICE NELSON
Assistant Professor of Nursing
Adelphi University

Contents

Clinical Perspectives in Nursing Research

RELEVANCE, SUFFERING, RECOVERY

The Relevance and Use of the Clinical Laboratory: NURSING STUDENTS' PERCEPTIONS

Geraldine Allerman & Mary Xenia Britten

THIS STUDY was conducted to discover how selected baccalaureate and associate degree nursing students perceived the relevance and use of the clinical laboratory as it pertained to their educational preparation for nursing practice. One purpose was to describe these perceptions as they relate to the development of selected professional and technical behaviors. Another was to identify the similarities and differences among the students' perceptions.

BACKGROUND AND RATIONALE

Key words in the study were defined as follows:

Relevance: " . . . the importance ascribed by an individual to selected aspects . . . of specific situations and of his activities and plans" (Schutz, 1973, p. 321). "A specific kind of relationship, one in which bearing or pertinence is shown" (Clayton, 1970, p. 134). One aspect of a situation is meaningful to the other. (The term is applied to the relationship described by the students between the information learned in the classroom and the activities practiced in the clinical laboratory.)

Clinical laboratory: "Those settings which provide the learner direct contact with recipients of nursing care" (Zungolo, 1972, p. 27).

There are many reasons why a study of this nature was needed. Because educators assume that the clinical laboratory is important as a setting in which students have the opportunity to practice nursing behaviors, it was necessary to consider its relevance to educational preparation for nursing practice. It is important for nursing educators to discover whether the aims

11

of the clinical laboratory are being achieved. Numerous studies have provided evidence that they are not.

For example, Zasowska (1967, p. 189) found that the clinical laboratory was used in an unquestioning fashion and was assumed by the faculty to be useful rather than determined as such. Recent studies of professional practice by Stokes (1977), Longman (1973), Tanner (1973), and Seedor indicated that graduates of baccalaureate programs were not exhibiting professional nursing behaviors. Whether students had the opportunity while in the clinical laboratory to learn the expected behaviors needed to be investigated.

Because data indicate that students influence their own socialization and thus determine in part the nature of the learning experience in the clinical setting (Zungolo, 1972, p. 238), it was essential to consult with students themselves. The student must see the relationship between theory presented in the classroom and the learning activity provided in the clinical laboratory. There must be a relationship between the behaviors practiced and learned in the clinical laboratory and the technical and professional behaviors expected of them as graduates. The students must perceive this relationship.

It was assumed (1) that the students would be able to evaluate and comment upon their preparation, (2) that content relating to the nursing behaviors would have been presented prior to the clinical laboratory experience, and (3) that the clinical laboratory provided opportunity for the student to develop nursing behaviors.

There were two limitations stated for this study. Lack of randomization and the size of the sample prevented generalization to all baccalaureate and associate degree nursing students. Use of a questionnaire limited the ability to control for the validity and depth of the responses.

Two concepts provided the framework for the study: the concept of relevance and that of professional and technical nursing practice.

Many educators, philosophers, sociologists, and phenomenologists have studied *relevance*. It must be remembered that relevance is "not an absolute property; nothing is either relevant or irrelevant in and of itself" (Scheffler, 1969, p. 764). It is the individual involved who determines what is of major importance and what is of minor importance. Each individual determines his own system of relevance. The steps or actions that one will pursue in life are directed toward one's goals and purposes, and these have been organized according to a system of relevance (Schutz, 1970, p. xiii).

Recently educators have stated that relevance influences the manner in which knowledge is ordered and retained (Bruner, 1971, p. xii; Appel, 1970, p. 85). Thomas F. Green developed a useful classification of relevance for educators. He distinguishes five categories of relevance, of which personal and programmatic provided the most value for this study (Green, 1969).

Personal relevance is concerned with the individual as a person—with what is meaningful to him and whether he has direct input into decisions made concerning him. *Programmatic relevance* is vocational or social and concerns the relevance or irrelevance of educational content to rather specific vocational goals.

Green further analyzes relevance in terms of the *relevance of means to ends*. This refers to the presence or absence of a "fit" between means and ends. Green identifies three types of relationships:

1. *Reasonable choice of means.* Means will be irrelevant to ends if the means chosen cannot be reasonably expected to achieve the desired ends. For example, if a student intends to master the elements of group dynamics, it would be irrelevant to study statistics; in such a case there is no "fit" of means to ends.

2. *Reliability of means chosen.* Means that appear to be relevant may turn out to be something different from what was anticipated. For example, a student wishing to learn group dynamics enrolls in a course entitled "Working with Groups," but the instructor spends the semester presenting Freud's theory of personality development; in this case the "fit" is only apparent.

3. *Relevant consequences of irrelevant means.* On the surface certain means appear irrelevant, yet turn out to be not only relevant but highly effective in arriving at desired ends.

For example, a student may learn the principles of group dynamics by participating in a seminar on Greek literature.

Nursing educators must ask these questions: Will the course instruction and clinical laboratory experience in the nursing curriculum assist the student to become a nurse? Are they relevant to nursing? Are the course content and the laboratory experience related and relevant to each other?

The second conceptual thrust of the study dealt with professional and technical nursing practice. *Models of professional and technical nurse performance*, encompassing behaviors ascribed by the literature to the two kinds of practice, were developed. Both models were validated or revised by three experts in nursing education.

Stokes' Model of Professional Nurse Performance was selected to serve as a basis for defining the behaviors expected of baccalaureate nursing students (Stokes, 1977, pp. 134-135). This model, derived from the literature, included the attributes of *knowledge base* and *autonomy of action*, with activities exemplifying each. For this study, these activities were adapted and expanded, following our own search of the literature on baccalaureate education in nursing and the role and functions of the professional nurse. Five activity categories were listed under the attribute of knowledge base (comprising 40 specific behaviors) and three under autonomy of action (16 behaviors) in the final model. It should be noted that certain behaviors were included in both the professional and technical models.

The Model of Technical Nurse Performance was developed in a similar manner. It was derived from the literature on associate degree education in nursing and the role and functions of the technical nurse. Eight activity categories were listed under knowledge base (30 behaviors) and seven under autonomy of action (34 behaviors). Although the literature states that the technical nurse provides care under the supervision of the professional nurse, within the scope of technical practice there are activities that are performed autonomously.

STUDY METHOD

Two structured three-part *questionnaires* were developed, one for associate degree nursing students and one for baccalaureate students. The complete questionnaires and models of nursing performance are presented in the authors' dissertation (1974).

Part I solicited background information about the students and was the same in both questionnaires.

Part II consisted of open-ended questions asking students to describe many aspects of their most recent clinical experience. Content was designed to relate to the behaviors in the appropriate model of nurse performance (the technical model for the associate degree students, the professional model for the baccalaureate students). The questions allowed the students to describe in their own words the *use* of the clinical laboratory.

Part III was designed to elicit students' views of the *relevance* of the clinical laboratory in relation to the nursing behaviors in the appropriate performance model. These were all listed, and for each one the students were requested (*a*) to indicate whether the *opportunity* existed for them to learn and practice the behavior and (*b*) to rate on a five-point scale how "*meaningful*" they believed the clinical laboratory to be as it pertained to learning and practicing the behavior. These items were followed by open-ended questions directed to *personal relevance*. The personal relevance items were identical in both questionnaires.

Reliability was built into each questionnaire by asking the same questions, slightly altered, in both Parts II and III and by including some similar questions within sections. Analysis of the responses revealed that the items were consistent. The instrument was submitted to the three nursing educators for content validation. All three agreed on its validity.

Nursing degree programs accredited by the National League for Nursing in metropolitan New York and New Jersey were invited to participate in the study. Six associate degree and five baccalaureate programs agreed to do so. Anonymity of each student and school was assured.

All participating students were in the last semester of their respective programs and were within a month of being graduated. Because the respondents would so soon assume the role of professional or technical nurse, it was felt that they should be cognizant of and should have had the opportunity to practice the behaviors ascribed to their respective roles. Also, they should be able to make discriminatory judgments regarding the relevance of the clinical laboratory.

The respondents were 276 associate degree and 163 baccalaureate nursing students. Because randomization was not used in the selection of the sample, generalizations could be made only to the sample group itself. The fact that some schools were willing to participate whereas others were not might have had a biasing influence on the findings.

The questionnaire data from Part II and the open-ended questions in Part III were subjected to content analysis utilizing the behaviors described in the models of technical and professional nurse performance as categories for analysis. All other items were analyzed by computer. The concepts of relevance in education and professional and technical nursing practice provided the framework for data analysis. Total frequency and the percentage of the response for each item were obtained.

RESULTS

Demographic data revealed that, although the majority of students in both types of programs were in the 21–25 year age group, the associate degree students were more heterogeneous, having representation in all age categories. Both groups were overwhelmingly female; however, there was a higher percentage of males in associate degree programs than in baccalaureate programs.

While many baccalaureate students selected their schools because of location, their main reason was the schools' reputation. The associate degree students chose their schools because of location.

The majority of the respondents had from one to five years of experience in health agencies prior to entering their respective programs. The most frequent position held was that of nursing aide.

Most of the students were currently employed in health agencies on a part-time basis. It was noteworthy that, whereas only two baccalaureate students cited practical nurse experience prior to program entrance, fifty-six stated that they were currently employed as practical nurses. It would appear that a large percentage obtained practical nurse licenses while learning to become professional nurses. This raises issues to be discussed later, regarding role identity and socialization.

From Part II of the questionnaire, which asked students to describe and discuss their most recent clinical experience in some detail, it was ascertained that the associate degree students were not engaged in practicing many of the behaviors attributed to knowledge base in the Model of Technical Nurse Performance: only nine of the thirty behaviors, or 30 per cent, were reportedly practiced by more than 50 per cent of the students. Because gathering data, assessing needs, developing plans to meet stated goals, and evaluating and revising plans are important activities the literature ascribes to technical nursing practice, one would expect students to be engaged in these activities to a greater degree than was reported.

With respect to autonomy of action, the second attribute examined, it was evident that the majority of the time spent by associate degree students in the clinical laboratory was devoted to daily hygienic care of the patient and nursing care appropriate to patients with common disorders. Positioning and ambulating patients were frequently cited, as well as assisting patients to meet nutritional needs. Psychosocial aspects of patient care, with provision for patients to ventilate feelings, were cited frequently by the students and evidently much weight was ascribed to them.

According to these students' descriptions, 50 per cent or more were engaged in learning only two, or 6 per cent, of the thirty-four selected behaviors associated with autonomy of action in the Model of Technical Nurse Performance. The behaviors that exemplified supervision and guidance of ancillary personnel were not manifest. Because these are behaviors the literature ascribes to technical nursing practice, one would expect the students to be engaged in these activities to a far greater degree than was reported.

The baccalaureate students in this study described knowledge base activities that related predominantly to gathering information and to providing nursing care that could be characterized as "routine" in nature. Nursing care plans existed but were often "in the head of the nurse" and rarely revised. Descriptions of patients' goals were vague, other than "the goal of the patient is to go home." Often the family was not included in the care even when student comments indicated that they were present. Evaluation of care seemed to be of a short-term nature. Few students noted results of patient laboratory data or tests in arriving at decisions for care.

With respect to autonomy of action, the baccalaureate students noted that they had had the leadership theory but had yet to put it into practice. Since they would be graduating within four weeks, one can only speculate as to when, if ever, they would have the practice opportunity.

There was surprising similarity evidenced between the associate degree and baccalaureate nursing students' use of clinical laboratory settings to learn and practice nursing behaviors. In both programs the students spent time collecting data on their patients, gave "AM care," and carried out treatments that were ordered. Psychosocial aspects of care were frequently cited by students in both groups and appeared to receive emphasis in the programs. Students in both programs indicated that they utilized various treatment modalities and that they charted and reported the patient's status. Few differences in the use of the clinical laboratory existed, other than that baccalaureate students reported experiences in public health agencies whereas associate degree students did not.

As previously noted, Part III of the questionnaire was designed to elicit students' perceptions of the *opportunities* to learn and practice selected behaviors in the clinical laboratory and the *relevance* of the clinical laboratory as a setting in which to do so. From the data both on knowledge base and on autonomy of action, it appeared that the associate degree nursing students in this study did perceive the laboratory as providing the opportunity to learn and practice the behaviors the literature ascribes to technical nursing practice. Also, they indicated that the laboratory was a "very meaningful" or "meaningful" setting in which to do so. They perceived it as a relevant means to attain the behaviors expected of them as practitioners. The exception relating to knowledge base was participation in evaluation of the patient's progress, and the one relating to autonomy was supervision of ancillary personnel in delivering care.

From the baccalaureate student data on knowledge base and autonomy of action, it appeared that these students also perceived the laboratory as providing the opportunity to learn and practice appropriate behaviors (those ascribed to professional nursing practice). And they also indicated that the laboratory was a "very meaningful" or "meaningful" setting in which to do so. They perceived it as a relevant means to attain the behaviors expected of them as professional practitioners. However, because of the number of students who responded negatively regarding behaviors related to data collection, implementation, and evaluation and revision of nursing care, further study is suggested. Also, many students indicated that they did not see the laboratory as providing opportunity to learn and practice many leadership behaviors.

While the responses in Part III revealed that the students perceived their situations as providing opportunity to learn and practice selected behaviors ascribed to their respective practice, the data from Part II indicated that they did not engage in many of them! Neither group engaged in data gathering, assessing, designing care plans, or evaluating and revising care plans to the depth the literature deems appropriate. Teaching and counseling patients and/or families received little or no emphasis. The behaviors associated with autonomous action were not evident. This is especially serious for baccalaureate students who are purported to be prepared for leadership roles.

Toward the end of their respective questionnaires, both groups were asked to respond to one set of ten questions designed to elicit more data regarding students' perceptions of the relevance of the clinical laboratory. These questions were formulated using Bruner's and Green's concepts of relevance in education.

The groups' responses were similar. They indicated that they would increase the amount of time spent in the clinical laboratory, that the laboratory was focused on meeting their individual learning needs, and that the time spent in the laboratory was predetermined by the faculty. Whereas the baccalaureate students indicated that the primary focus was on them (the learners), the associate degree students responded that it was on caring for patients.

The respondents indicated that there were objectives for their clinical nursing course, objectives specific to the clinical laboratory, and specific objectives for each clinical laboratory experience; that the objectives were formulated by the faculty but that they had their own personal objectives for each clinical laboratory experience; and that even when they had achieved the objectives, they were still required to participate in the laboratory.

It is unfortunate that such a high percentage of students stated that the faculty formulated the objectives and determined the time spent in the clinical laboratory. Learning theory states that the individual must be considered in planning curricula. The objectives must take into consideration the student's abilities, interests, and past life experiences. He must find the experience meaningful and satisfying in order to be motivated to learn.

A concern of *personal relevance,* in terms of Green's concept (1969), is whether the individual has direct input into decisions that are made concerning him. If the student is to perceive the clinical laboratory as a meaningful setting in which to learn, he must contribute to the formulation of the clinical laboratory objectives. The student and faculty member must collaborate in order to assure the student meaningful learning experiences. This is crucial in both programs. The associate degree students come into their programs with a wide variety of life experiences and represent many age groups. What is relevant for one student may not be relevant for another.

Although the baccalaureate students are a more homogeneous group, they also have individual differences that must be considered in planning their learning experiences. If they are to be encouraged to practice leadership behaviors, one should certainly expect them to have input into their learning experiences. They should be cognizant of their learning needs and encouraged to design and implement plans to meet them.

One also questions why students who have achieved the objectives are still required to participate in the clinical laboratory. If a student has successfully met the objective, one concludes that he has learned the specified behavior. If the behavior has been learned, requiring the student to remain in the setting may result in meaningless repetition and/or miseducation.

It should be noted that approximately 90 per cent of both student groups stated that they had their own personal objectives for each clinical laboratory experience. Ascertaining the students' personal goals would be an enlightening study.

In order to ascertain the activities the students perceived themselves performing in the clinical laboratory, they were asked to list the four activities they performed most often and the four performed least often.

The baccalaureate group indicated that they most often gave medications, gave hygienic care ("AM care"), engaged in nurse/patient interactions, and ascertained vital signs. The associate degree students responded that they gave hygienic care, gave medications, ascertained vital signs, and made beds.

The baccalaureate students least often performed catheterizations, engaged in collaborative actions, conducted nursing rounds, and led conferences with nurses and other staff. The associate degree respondents least often performed catheterizations, suctioned patients, gave medications, and monitored infusions. The associate degree group listed administering medications as an activity performed most often and also as an activity performed least often.

One is again struck by the similarities between the groups. Three of the four activities listed as performed most often are the same for both groups. Except for catheterizations, the groups listed different activities for those performed least often. It should also be noted that three of the four activities listed as performed least often by baccalaureate students are activities associated with leadership. This reinforces the other indications that baccalaureate students are not learning and practicing the autonomous activities the literature ascribes to professional nursing practice. The question also arises as to whether the respective educational institutions are in fact preparing different practitioners. The data suggest that the students from baccalaureate and associate degree programs are engaged in the same activities.

Because the literature states that the clinical laboratory is the place in which classroom information is put into practice (Infante, 1971, p. 16), students were asked whether they were able to put information presented in their most recent class into practice in the clinical laboratory later during the current week. Only 55 per cent of the baccalaureate students and 44 per cent of the associate degree students stated that they were able to do so. This was the situation as perceived by the students. However, the reality of the situation may have involved an even lower percentage of students putting prior-presented classroom theory into practice the same week. In many instances, careful comparison of the kinds of information listed with the report of performed activities as described in Part II of the questionnaires indicated that putting the listed classroom information into practice would have been inappropriate in the described clinical situation (e.g., utilizing chemotherapeutic principles of neoplasm therapy would have been inappropriate in caring for a patient who has sustained a traumatic injury).

Additional student comments and/or suggestions regarding the clinical laboratory indicated clearly that the two groups had similar concerns. In both groups a majority expressed the desire to increase the amount of time spent in the clinical laboratory. They voiced apprehension and lack of confidence in assuming their expected roles and in performing "procedures." Both groups noted that caring for patients only once was inadequate for establishing continuity of care, developing nursing goals, and evaluating and revising nursing care plans. They made comments about not being given adequate responsibility while in the clinical laboratory.

Both groups cited favorably the availability of their instructors; but they also mentioned that the nursing staffs in the clinical settings often "misinterpreted the roles and the nature of [students'] academic programs." The students indicated there was a lack of communication between them and the nursing staffs in the health agencies.

With respect to differences, the baccalaureate students were more concerned with the individuality of their learning experiences and expressed the desire that more independent study be incorporated into their programs. They made more frequent reference to the educational purposes of the clinical laboratory experience. They offered suggestions for what they viewed as improvements in the clinical laboratory experience and emphatically expressed the desire for a voice in decision making.

Various data, then, suggested that from the students' perspective the clinical laboratory could be made more personally relevant. It is evident that students felt they had little, if any, input into decisions concerning their clinical laboratory experiences. Faculty formulated the objectives and determined the time spent in the clinical laboratory. One of the most frequent comments of the students was that they wished "a voice in decision making."

Programmatic relevance is another concept that provides a framework for analysis. This, as Green (1969) defines it, is "relevance or irrelevance of educational content to rather specific vocational goals." Although the students of this study perceived the clinical laboratory as relevant, the data clearly indicated that they were not engaged in many of the activities the literature ascribes to their respective practice. This was especially true of the independent activities ascribed to a professional nurse. It is also clear from students' responses that course content and laboratory experience were not related to each other. This was evident when one compared the classroom points listed with the activities in which students reported they were engaged on a specific day in the clinical laboratory. It was also made clear by students frequently commenting that faculty should "try to correlate class with the clinical experience; the lab is integral—make it so." The similarity of the activities in which both groups were engaged raises questions as to whether, indeed, two types of practitioners are being prepared.

The findings of the study may also be considered in terms of Green's (1969) criteria for the *relevance of means to ends.*

With respect to the relationship he calls "reasonable choice of means," it was found that the students viewed the means chosen (the clinical laboratory) as appropriate and relevant even though the ends (learning appropriate nursing behaviors) were not achieved.

Concerning "reliability of means chosen," the data indicate that although the clinical laboratory appeared relevant as a means to learn and practice technical and professional nursing behaviors, it did not in fact provide the means appropriate to such behaviors. The means chosen turned out to be different from what was assumed.

From the data one may speculate that the students' "workships" (their employment in health agencies, unrelated to their educational programs) might provide a means that appears irrelevant but turns out to be highly effective in arriving at desired ends. In other words, one would not anticipate that employment as a nursing aide or practical nurse would lead to learning of behaviors expected of professional or technical nurses, yet such employment may indeed achieve that end. Green calls this "relevant consequences of irrelevant means."

CONCLUSIONS AND IMPLICATIONS

Although definitive judgments regarding the reality of the situation cannot be made without observational studies, the following conclusions have been drawn: Both groups of nursing students perceived the clinical laboratory as a setting that provided the opportunity to learn and practice the selected behaviors associated with knowledge base and autonomy of action as described in the models of technical and professional nurse performance. And they viewed it as a "meaningful" setting in which to do so. In short, the respondents perceived the clinical laboratory as a relevant means to attain the behaviors expected of them as practitioners.

However, from the students' descriptions of their activities, it was evident that they were not engaged in learning and practicing the behaviors ascribed to their respective practice. The associate degree students spent the majority of their clinical time administering daily hygienic care to patients with common problems. The baccalaureate students were predominantly engaged in data-gathering activities related to providing nursing care of "routine" nature. There was little evidence of leadership behavior.

Information presented in the classroom was not correlated with clinical laboratory experience. Also, the laboratory experience was not found to be personally relevant. Although the clinical laboratory has the potential for being programmatically relevant, in this study it was not found to be so. In spite of the fact that the means chosen appeared relevant, in many instances the "fit" between means and ends was only apparent. From the students' descriptions, it was evident that the clinical laboratory did not provide the means to learn and practice the selected technical and professional nursing behaviors.

The findings of this study hold many implications for nursing education and nursing service. Because of the many similarities in the activities being practiced by associate degree and baccalaureate students in the clinical laboratory, one can anticipate that without appropriate intervention the present blurring of technical and professional roles and functions will continue and perhaps increase. If, prior to graduation, students are not engaged in practicing the behaviors ascribed to their practice, one cannot expect them to exhibit these behaviors as practitioners.

Questions are raised as to the student's identity. Whereas associate degree students requested more leadership skills, baccalaureate students asked for more technical skills. One must ask whether nursing students are cognizant of the roles and functions ascribed to technical and professional practice. If they are, do they identify with their respective roles? If not, this will also contribute to the blurring of roles.

Since the students perceived the laboratory as providing the opportunity, one must ask why the students were not engaged in learning and practicing the selected behaviors. What factors operate to prevent them from doing so? Are faculty members cognizant of the behaviors? Do they teach to them? If they are and they do, are the clinical laboratory experiences designed to foster them? What is it about the public health experience that allows for practice of more professional behaviors?

Nursing educators must note that half the students indicated that the primary focus of the clinical laboratory was on caring for the patient rather than on them, the learners. This implied that the emphasis was on patient care rather than on student learning. Does this signify that the clinical laboratory was utilized to enable the student to "do to learn" rather than to "learn to do"?

Students' statements that the staff of the service agencies were not clear regarding the students' roles and academic programs implied a lack of communication between school faculty and the staff of the service institution. Data also indicated that the staff in many agencies did not utilize care plans, hold patient conferences, conduct nursing rounds, or communicate among themselves. This signified that the nursing staff in these agencies were not exhibiting the behaviors described in the models of technical and professional nurse performance. They were not fulfilling their roles and functions as described in the literature.

Because the clinical laboratory is seen to be a necessary component of a nursing curriculum and perceived as meaningful by the students, it is essential that it be utilized appropriately. From the data it is evident that measures must be taken to ensure the relevance of the clinical laboratory.

RECOMMENDATIONS

In light of the findings, the following are recommendations for nursing faculty:

1. Design the clinical laboratory experience so that it will be more personally relevant for students. Faculty should consult with students in formulating objectives for each laboratory experience. In fact, the entire clinical laboratory should be planned collaboratively with the student. Individualization of the learning experience is essential.

2. Identify clearly the technical and professional behaviors expected of students upon graduation and design the curriculum accordingly. These behaviors must be taught and fostered throughout the respective programs.

3. Inform the students of the nursing roles and functions attributed to both technical and professional nursing practice. Practitioners from both types of programs will be employed in the same setting.

4. Examine carefully the students' learning experiences in the clinical laboratory. Faculty must ensure that the student will have the opportunity to practice desired behaviors and

provide encouragement to do so. In order to accomplish this, the faculty must consider not only patient assignment but also the time of day in which the student is in the laboratory. If always assigned on a one-time basis, it is difficult (if not impossible) for the student to learn to evaluate the patient's response to therapy. Faculty must provide greater flexibility in the use of the clinical laboratory. Assignments cannot be made on a time and place basis. The students' objectives must dictate the learning experience. For example, if attaining a psychomotor skill is the objective, frequent short periods in the laboratory are appropriate.

5. Explore all instructional methods in assisting students to learn the practice of nursing. Simulation, role-playing, videotapes, computers, and case studies may be utilized to assist students to learn to implement, evaluate, and revise the plan of care they have formulated with the data they gathered. For example, a programmed manikin may be utilized to assist the student in learning to make care decisions based on a knowledge of how patients generally respond to therapy. This also provides the student the opportunity to test theory in a controlled setting.

6. Correlate practice more closely with theory.

7. Design baccalaureate curricula to emphasize leadership behavior. Leadership principles must be taught at the time the student enters the program and reinforced throughout.

8. Design learning experiences in light of students' individual differences.

9. Attend inservice education programs designed to assist faculty to learn to utilize the clinical and college laboratories more effectively.

10. Communicate more effectively with health agency nursing personnel.

The following recommendations are for nursing students, who should:

1. Be given a greater voice in making decisions which affect them. Their active participation not only enhances their learning, it also results in the educational program becoming more relevant.

2. Assume a greater role in designing curriculum, evaluating courses, and participating in committees.

3. Identify more clearly the goals toward which they are working.

4. Formulate personal objectives for each clinical laboratory session.

The nursing curriculum should be:

1. Evaluated in light of the behaviors ascribed to technical and professional nursing practice in order to ascertain whether the students' courses of study enhance their learning.

2. Designed in baccalaureate programs so that leadership behaviors will be taught early and fostered throughout the student's program.

3. Designed in associate degree programs so that the behaviors ascribed to autonomy of action in technical nursing practice may be taught early and fostered throughout.

Because upon graduation these students will be employed in service agencies, agency personnel should:

1. Become cognizant of the philosophies of baccalaureate and associate degree nursing programs so that the agency can have more realistic expectations of its nursing personnel.

2. Evaluate their present nursing staff practices to ascertain whether they demonstrate the behaviors the literature ascribes to technical and professional nursing practice.

3. Review the nursing staff job descriptions to ascertain whether they are consistent with behaviors ascribed to technical and professional nursing practice.

4. Provide a setting in which nursing staff will be encouraged to practice the selected nursing behaviors.

5. Design an inservice education program to teach and foster the selected behaviors attributed to technical and professional practice. Assuming these behaviors are desired, nursing service agencies must assist their staff to learn and practice them. (It is envisaged that nursing inservice programs would teach the respective behaviors to recent graduates only until there is evidence that the educational programs have done so. And even if the desired behaviors have been taught, inservice training must assist the new graduate in further developing them. The recent graduate of either program is a beginning practitioner and at this juncture socialization is not complete.)

6. Improve communication between the service agency staff and the college nursing faculty.

7. Participate in college committees so as to increase cooperation and communication between academic and service agencies.

8. Allow nursing students and faculty more freedom to engage in laboratory activities designed to meet students' learning needs.

The findings in this study have raised many questions that suggest recommendations for nursing research:

1. Replicate the study, increasing the sample size and utilizing randomization.

2. Conduct a study in which students respond to the questionnaire after investigators have observed them in the clinical laboratory.

3. Conduct a study in which the students' and faculty's perceptions of the relevance and use of the clinical laboratory are elicited simultaneously.

4. Conduct an observational study to ascertain the activities in which nursing students are engaged in the clinical laboratory.

5. Conduct an observational study to ascertain the activities in which nursing students are engaged in both the classroom and the clinical laboratory.

6. Conduct an observational study utilizing the models of technical and professional nurse performance to ascertain the activities in which nursing practitioners are engaged in service agencies.

7. Design a study to identify the factors that might militate against students' engaging in the selected behaviors attributed to their respective practice.

8. Investigate baccalaureate nursing students' employment as practical nurses while they are studying to become professional nurses.

9. Conduct a study to determine the factors that enhance baccalaureate student performance of selected professional behaviors in the public health setting.

10. Conduct a study to determine nursing students' personal goals as they are engaged in learning the practice of nursing.

Students in general often complain that curricula are not designed in light of their interests and purposes. A legitimate desire of nursing students is that they be assisted in bridging the gap between theory that is presented and its ultimate use in *nursing practice*. As Donald Sharpe says, discussing the importance of professional laboratory experience in teacher education (1956, p. 221): "Theory without experience is baseless and idle speculation. Practice without theoretical base is blind, unintelligent and acquiescent."

Although the nursing students in this study perceived the clinical laboratory as being relevant to the learning and practice of selected nursing behaviors, a clear discrepancy was revealed when they described the activities in which they actually engaged. It behooves nursing faculty to further study the use of the clinical laboratory. For, as Jonas Soltis has said (1968, p. 51): "When all is said and done about the process of educating, it is ultimately the actual result of the process which is left to evidence our success or failure."

REFERENCES

Allerman, Geraldine, & Britten, Mary X. "Nursing Students' Perceptions of the Relevance and Use of the Clinical Laboratory in Learning the Practice of Nursing." Ed.D. dissertation, Teachers College, Columbia University, 1974.

Appel, Michael W. "Relevance and Curriculum: A Study in Phenomenological Sociology of Knowledge." Ed.D dissertation, Teachers College, Columbia University, 1970.

Bruner, Jerome S. *The Relevance of Education*. New York: W. W. Norton, 1971.

Clayton, A. Stafford. "Education and Some Moves toward a Value Methodology." In *Theories of Value and Problems of Education*. Edited by Philip G. Smith. Urbana: Univ. of Illinois Press, 1970.

Green, Thomas F. "The Concept of Relevance in Education." Paper presented at the American Philosophical Association Symposium, New York, December 29, 1969.

Infante, Mary Sue. "The Laboratory Concept in Baccalaureate Education in Nursing." Ed.D. dissertation, Teachers College, Columbia University, 1971.

Longman, Alice J. "Professional Nurse Behavior Demonstrated in Caring for a Patient with Chronic Obstructive Pulmonary Disease." Ed.D. dissertation, Teachers College, Columbia University, 1973.

Scheffler, Israel. "Reflections on Educational Relevance." *Journal of Philosophy* 66 (November 1969).

Schutz, Alfred. *Studies in Phenomenological Philosophy:* Vol. III of *Collected Papers.* Edited by I. Schutz. The Hague: Martinus Nijhoff, 1970.

———. *On Phenomenology and Social Relations.* Edited by Helmut R. Wagner. Chicago: Univ. of Chicago Press, 1973.

Seedor, Marie M. "Preliminary Inquiry into the Level of Nursing Practiced by the Professional Nurse." Pilot study funded by the National Institute of Health.

Sharpe, Donald M. "Professional Laboratory Experiences." In *Teacher Education for a Free People.* Edited by Donald P. Cottrell. Oneonta, N.Y.: American Association of Colleges for Teacher Education, 1956.

Soltis, Jonas F. *An Introduction to the Analysis of Educational Concepts.* Reading, Mass.: Addison-Wesley, 1968.

Stokes, Shirlee Ann. "Selected Professional Behaviors Exhibited in Clinical Practice." In *Present Realities/Future Imperatives in Nursing Education.* Edited by M. Louise Fitzpatrick. New York: Teachers College Press, 1977.

Tanner, Sr. Gloria Ann. "Heart Failure Patients and the Coronary Care Unit." Ed.D. dissertation, Teachers College, Columbia University, 1973.

Zasowska, Sr. Aloise Anne. "A Descriptive Survey of Significant Factors in the Clinical Laboratory Experience in Baccalaureate Education for Nursing." Ed.D. dissertation, Teachers College, Columbia University, 1967.

Zungolo, Eileen. "A Systems Analysis of Clinical Laboratory Experiences in Baccalaureate Nursing Education." Ed.D. dissertation, Teachers College, Columbia University, 1972.

Critique

Sr. Aloise Anne Zasowska

THE TASK of integrating knowledge to be expressed as an action behavior has plagued philosophers, frustrated social scientists, and eluded professional practitioners both in educational circles and in the research arena over the years. For, the expression of effective performance in the form of demonstrable behavior requires an integration of knowledge buttressed by a well-conceived perception of role and function expectations.

I trust I am not presumptuous in stating that my audience undoubtedly shares with me the view that a thorough and probing review of the pervading issues raised by the outcomes of Dr. Allerman's and Dr. Britten's study can be given only a very cursory analysis during this brief conference time. However, I wish to emphasize at the outset that the data, however limited for purposes of generalization, cannot be discounted as inconsequential; to the contrary, they must indeed evoke a feeling of uneasiness in nursing educators and once again raise questions in the technical/professional domains of the profession. The discomforting picture painted by the data and the outcomes of the study may, due to intervening variables, present some problematic *non sequiturs*. However, an attempt at analysis of unaccounted for variables may well result in the neglect of broad and far-reaching implications of the study.

The study of the perception of relevance is not only involved but intriguing. Results of the study reveal that "the respondents perceived the clinical laboratory as a relevant means to attain the behaviors expected of them as practitioners. However, from the students' descriptions of their activities, it was evident that they were not engaged in learning and practicing the behaviors ascribed to their respective practice." This raises issues related not only to the ordering of the clinical setting but more perhaps to the causality in behavior and questions about behavior mechanisms. Methodologies and designs for systems organization leading to behavior models as means to achieve relevance need to be considered. Is it the *laboratory,* or is it a form of *organization,* that is required to effectuate the reproduction in present time of a behavior constructed on a data base of concepts and past experiences? Must we not rather address this question: If behavior is a process that involves responses based in perception, should not the educator concentrate efforts on ordering learning experiences previously *validated* on the basis of what *is perceived* as appropriate and adequate, rather than *postulate* what is *to be perceived* and therefore what the consequent behavior will be?

Should the analysis of this study direct us to persist in asking, "Does the student perceive the clinical laboratory to be relevant?" Or should we not look to the compelling need for the deliberate construction of organized systems for expected behavior outcomes, with perception of relevance both directed and assured?

Rather than *providing* laboratory experiences, the need may be to understand how to diagnose and construct experience, how to facilitate action, and how to monitor the behavior while simultaneously achieving educational goals. The learner must be the originator rather than the receptor, active rather than passive, responsible and responsive rather than accepting of the environment and the experience itself. If there is *knowledge* of expected behavior and its consequences, what interferes with *behaving* as expected? Factors affecting knowledge and *behaving* may need to be the subject of investigation.

Drs. Britten and Allerman found "that the clinical laboratory did not provide the means to learn and practice the selected technical and professional nursing behaviors." Does the answer lie in the *provision* of laboratory experiences through placement in settings that in truth can hardly eventuate in goal-directed behavior? Or should not our effort be directed at the development and adoption of a theory of action and a process of learning as the basis of professional/technical practice? We want not a recitation of a theory, but rather a defined theory of what constitutes and results in the expected behaviors of nursing practice.

The outcomes of the study beg the question: If nursing behaviors (professional/technical) are definitive in nature, and if these defined behaviors constitute terminal objectives of the nursing curriculum, then is it a matter of perceived relevance of the laboratory experience, or is it not rather a question of whether the learning process has been *constructed* to achieve desired objectives?

Again, Drs. Allerman and Britten state: "Both groups of students perceived the clinical laboratory as a setting that provided the opportunity to learn and practice the selected behaviors associated with knowledge base and autonomy of action as described in the models of technical and professional nurse performance." Yet the activities they performed did not *engage* them in the selected behaviors made possible through the clinical laboratory.

Where—what—is the missing link? Are we justified in faulting the structure of the laboratory experience? Is it not perhaps the conceptual framework of the behavior process? Or is this evidence of what Argyris and Schon (1974, p. viii) describe in their book *Theory in Practice* as a dichotomy between *espoused theories* (those that describe and justify behavior) and *theories-in-use* (those that govern our actions and contribute to specific constancies)?

According to Argyris and Schon (pp. 6–7), "When someone is asked how he would behave under certain circumstances, the answer he usually gives is his espoused theory of action for that situation. This is the theory to which he gives allegiance, and which, upon request, he communicates to others. However, the theory that actually governs his actions is his theory-in-use, which may or may not be compatible with his espoused theory; furthermore, the individual may or may not be aware of the incompatibility of the two theories."

Perhaps the need is to direct energy at researching and identifying a theory of practice consisting of a set of interrelated theories of action which will specify for the situations under study the actions that will yield intended consequences. This theory of action will need to address itself to the theory-in-use and the espoused theory.

In education for nursing practice, the requisite may be the internalization of a theory of action and its translation into actual behavior with congruence between the espoused theory and the theory-in-use. Further, faculty will need to be aware of their own theory-in-use and will need to identify the learner's theory-in-use, which may not only be the *modus operandi* but may indeed be an obstacle to learning.

This study and several other investigations have centered on whether students *learn or do not learn* in clinical laboratory; the outcomes are usually similar and not very comforting. Perhaps it is time to turn to theory building for professional practice. This will require practitioners with special competence related to diagnosis, to the generation and testing of solutions, and to the experience of personal causality in implementing the proposed solutions.

It may be the prompting of caution which, in my view, these investigators reflect in a rather "soft touch" approach in their recommendations. Their directives to faculty say things like this: (1) design clinical laboratory experiences for relevance; (2) identify expected behaviors; (3) inform students of roles and functions; (4) examine students' learning experiences; . . . . I would say *(with emphasis and without equivocation):* Educating students for practice—be it technical or professional—requires competent teachers at the forefront of nursing: teachers who are secure enough to recognize their responsibility for instruction and who are not threatened by the lack of consensus about nursing behavior; faculty skilled in helping students to *learn* expected behaviors through direct experience; educators skilled in knowledge of the learning process and in its utilization in the acquisition of *behavior;* practitioners skilled at being reflective about their actions and capable of developing theories of effective practice.

The questions persist: Who are the role models for the *behaviors* the students strive to adopt? Is there congruence between the espoused theories and the theories-in-use of the practitioner models in the field? Is the clinical experience truly integrated into the curriculum?

The onus is on the faculty—educators/practitioners—who

are competent in surfacing conflicts and incongruities in their fields; faculty whose sense of self-esteem and their intellectual integrity are high enough that they can admit the differences between what they teach and the practice the student learns; faculty who are strong enough to invite confrontation between what they teach and what is practiced. With obsolete or nonexistent consensual technical theory, it will be especially important to encourage the exploration of the underlying value conflicts that exist where professional activities are in transition. Few changes will be made in education or in practice unless faculties, students, and practitioners become more aware of their espoused interpersonal theories and their interpersonal theories-in-use.

The clinical laboratory experience must be the *process*— not the setting—wherein behavior occurs in directly observable categories, the *process* for examining inferences and testing hypotheses for continued feedback into the process. The laboratory as *process* must focus on double-loop learning, which involves changing of the governing variables of the experience: *learning* that is concerned with the surfacing and resolution of conflict rather than with its suppression; willingness to change the field of constancy and allow change to fan out over one's whole system of theories-in-use. In this process the learner will identify and express his theory-in-use in such a way that he feels responsible for it and does not attribute his behavior to the structure of the simulation but to his personal causation; in this process the learner will identify the governing variables of his behavior and explore the immediate and long-term consequences of his behavior on the client.

Dr. Mildred Montag in her pointedly poignant treatise *Where Is Nursing Going?* (1975, p. 8) claims that only "*statesmen* can lead us out of the confusion of the day." Drs. Britten and Allerman voice a crying need for faculty to bridge "the gap between theory that is presented and its ultimate use in *nursing practice*."

I say: Let us search out our statesmen and begin bridging the gap by building a theory of practice, and let us then design the *laboratory process* for its application.

Let us keep in mind what Camus says: "For a thought to

change the world, it must first change the life of the man who carries it. It must become an example."

REFERENCES

Argyris, Chris, & Schon, Donald A. *Theory in Practice: Increasing Professional Effectiveness.* (Washington, D.C.: Jossey-Bass, 1974).
Montag, Mildred L. *Where Is Nursing Going?* New York: NLN, 1975.

Nurses' Inferences of Suffering: THE EFFECTS OF NURSE-PATIENT SIMILARITY AND VERBALIZATIONS OF DISTRESS

Marilyn T. Oberst

BACKGROUND AND RATIONALE

GIVEN THE personal, private nature of pain and suffering, and the lack of general, agreed-upon definitions, judging whether another individual is in pain and the extent of his suffering is a potentially complex nursing task. It involves selecting appropriate cues from those available, measuring the selected cues against some predetermined standard, and reaching a conclusion by inference. We have considerable information on what experiences patients view as painful and under what circumstances they do so. But we know relatively little about the way in which nurses define pain and suffering, or about the extent to which they accept or reject (or, for that matter, are even aware of) those operational definitions available to them in the current nursing literature.

The primary purpose of this study was to determine the relationship between the degree of patients' suffering inferred by the nurse and the extent to which patient and nurse have similar characteristics of age and social class, and whether any alteration of this relationship occurs when patients verbally express their own suffering. Two secondary purposes were to determine the relative importance of cues used by nurses in determining the degree of another's suffering, and to explore nurses' personal definitions of suffering.

Clinical studies of pain and pain-related behavior emphasize the degree to which individuals may vary in their response patterns. An individual's ethnic background, cultural milieu, and personality traits influence definition, behavioral response, and coping style (Zborowski, 1952, 1969; Jacox & Stewart, 1973; Lynn & Eysenck, 1961). A person's subjective assessment of his own discomfort depends largely on his own criteria, and it is not necessarily related to the magnitude of the stimulus (Copp, 1974; Petrie, 1967, pp. 16-26).

Complaints of distress are powerful help-seeking mechanisms (Szasz, 1959, pp. 982-999; Szasz, 1957, pp. 82-104; Gonda, 1962), not usually invoked until distress is quite severe. Under such circumstances, patients who complain of distress do so with the expectation that relief will be forthcoming (Graffam, 1970; Jacox & Stewart, 1973). The evidence regarding nurse response to patients' distress is limited, but suggests that although nurses believe they should be able to tell when suffering is present, the single most salient cue is probably the patient's statement of distress (Graffam, 1970). Nurses have also been shown to have preconceived ideas and expectations about the degrees of suffering associated with various diagnoses and prognoses, and to have difficulty dealing with behaviors that deviate from the expected trajectory (Glaser & Strauss, 1965, 1968; Hackett, 1971; Strauss, Fagerhaugh, & Glaser, 1974).

Studies of the inferential processes used by nurses in determining the state of a patient suggest that cue selection may be largely intuitive (Hammond et al., 1967). Consistent patterns of cue utilization among groups of nurses have not been identified (Hammond et al., 1966a,b,c). One series of investigations found a number of factors to be related to the degree of suffering nurses believed patients to be experiencing. The major nurse characteristic identified was cultural or ethnic background, while the salient patient characteristics associated with differences in degree of suffering inferred included diagnosis, age, and social class (Davitz & Pendleton, 1969; Baer, Davitz, & Lieb, 1970; Lenburg, Glass, & Davitz, 1970; Lenburg, Burnside, & Davitz, 1970).

Nurses are aware of the real status differences that may exist between themselves and their patients; such awareness influences the number and type of interactions engaged in by the nurse. Interactions that threaten prestige are generally avoided, and there is a tendency to invoke the ideal of patient equality when client-caretaker social distance is greater. Nurses have been shown to interact more readily at their own middle class level and to have difficulty establishing relationships with patients above or below themselves in social class (King, 1962;

Segal, 1964; Weiss, 1968, p. 205). Attempts of patients to exert authority and autonomy may be perceived as ego-threatening to the nurse, with consequent reduction in the feelings of warmth and compassion engendered (Segal, 1964).

Classification of patients as "good" or "bad" does occur, and it may be directly related to the way in which the individual copes with suffering. Liked patients are those who suffer quietly and nobly, while disliked patients are apt to be chronic complainers who constantly seek attention (Ekdawi, 1967; Blaylock, 1970). Studies of helping behavior outside the health care situation suggest that the incidence of actions designed to reduce suffering may be related both to the kind of distress signal given by the victim and to the helper's perceived ability to alter the victim's fate (Yakimovich & Saltz, 1971; Lerner & Simmons, 1966; Baron, 1970).

CONCEPTUAL FRAMEWORK

The task of clinical inference is a cognitive process that leads to nursing action (Kelly, 1964a). It requires that the nurse infer, on the basis of the data presented by the patient, his impalpable, uncertain state, relying almost entirely on her own perceptual processes (Hammond, 1966) and utilizing a variety of subjective and objective informational cues, not all of which are equally relevant in all situations.

Kelly has defined clinical inference as requiring a face-to-face clinician/client relationship (Kelly, 1964a). For the purposes of this study, however, the inferential process was defined more broadly, and subjects were required to make judgments from written information about patients without the opportunity to seek additional data. The subjects' task was seen as one of deductive inference, a reasoning from prior generalizations to current instances. The assumption that such prior generalizations exist is based, in part, on Kelly's finding that individual nurses demonstrated consistency in the use of their own systems during the process of deriving inferences from available data (Kelly, 1964b). Such generalizations may have been arrived at through earlier induction, resulting in theoretical or empirical generalizations, or they may exist as stereotypes or intuitions. No attempt was made to isolate the source of these generalizations.

Shared social group membership can enhance the desire to engage in helping behaviors (Hornstein, 1972) and can produce greater accuracy of impression formation and increased ability to perceive and interpret expressive cues (Brown, 1965, pp. 640-646). This suggests that systematic variations in cue utilization and subsequent inference may exist as a function of client/caretaker similarities.

Insufficient empirical evidence existed to predict the exact nature or direction of the effect of nurse/patient similarities upon the degree of suffering inferred, or the relationship between a patient's verbalization of distress and the nurse's interpretation of that verbalization in the form of an inference of suffering. All hypotheses advanced for testing were therefore general and non-directional.

METHODOLOGY

Research Design: Although the general problem of nursing inference is clearly a clinical issue, a non-clinical setting, using written data to describe clinical situations, was used. Hammond and Kelly concluded after extensive clinical study that the complexity of the clinical setting precluded access to cue utilization behavior and recommended use of paper-and-pencil tests (Hammond et al., 1966a). The inference section of the study utilized repeated measures in a questionnaire format and followed the prototype designed by Davitz and Pendleton (1969). A basic assumption was that the process of drawing an inference of suffering from written data is similar to the cognitive process involved in making such an inference in the clinical setting. Lack of redundant or supporting information for verification of cues was recognized as a limitation.

Instrument: Two preliminary studies were undertaken to select diagnostic categories and verbal content which, in isolation, conveyed a moderate degree of suffering. Age, social class, verbalization or its absence, sex, and diagnosis were then systematically varied in a series of 108 written descriptions of patients; these descriptions were the items in the inference section of the questionnaire. Subjects read each item and indicated on a seven-point scale ranging from 0 (no suffering) to 6 (very severe suffering) the degree of suffering they believed the patient to be experiencing. A reliability estimate of .87 was obtained in pilot testing.

The second portion of the instrument presented subjects with a list of cues (facial expression, diagnosis, position and movements, vocalization, . . .) which they were asked to rank in order of importance in determining the degree of another's suffering. Finally the subjects, who had been told at the outset to use their own definition of suffering, were asked to write out that definition.

Subjects: An available population of nurses, in clinical practice at a single community hospital and closely resembling the national averages in age, education, and marital status, was pre-stratified into three age groups. Random sampling techniques were employed, and the final sample consisted of 153 nurses. Subjects' social class (SES) was determined on the basis of self-ratings.

FINDINGS

Mean scores (inferred suffering ratings on the 0–6 scale) were computed across items for each subject, and specific hypotheses relating to nurse characteristics were tested with analysis of variance. Subscores for various item types were used to compare responses to various patient characteristics. The mean score across items was 3.0963, just above the midpoint (moderate suffering) on the scale used. The range of means was from 1.50 to 4.23.

Table I shows means and *F* scores for the major nurse variables. A hypothesized relationship between nurse age and degree of suffering inferred was not supported. A similar hypothesis relating to the nurse's self-perceived social status was supported, with high SES subjects inferring less suffering than their low SES counterparts. No differences in mean scores were attributable to the nurse's education level, years of experience, area of specialization, work status, or marital status.

TABLE I

Mean Inferred Suffering Scores, Standard Deviations, and F Scores Among Nurse Subjects by Age and Social Class

Nurse Characteristic	N	Mean Score	Standard Deviation	F Score	Significance Level
Age					
Young	53	3.048	.52		
Mid-age	48	3.005	.50		
Older	51	3.233	.56		
				2.6559	N.S.
Social Class					
Low	53	3.224	.56		
High	100	3.029	.51		
				4.7649	p<.05

Hypotheses positing that patient age, social class, and the presence or absence of a verbalized distress signal would influence the degree of suffering were all supported. Table II gives a breakdown of means and F scores for various patient characteristics. The oldest group of patients were judged to suffer more than young or middle-aged ones. Of the three social classes described, middle class patients were seen as suffering less than those above or below them in class. Greater suffering was consistently inferred for those patients who verbalized distress. (See also Figures 1, 2, and 3.) The items containing verbalizations were further broken down into those representing general complaint statements and those in which relief was requested. Although the mean difference was small, a significantly higher mean score was found for patients who requested relief.

The control variables of patient sex and diagnosis were also examined. Sex was found to have no significant effect on the inferences made. Patient diagnosis markedly influenced the degree of suffering inferred. The six diagnoses were subjected to Scheffé contrasts and the following relationship emerged: the degree of suffering inferred for { post-op polypectomy > abscess of leg > hematoma > phlebitis > pneumonia > otitis media. } This suggests that ambulatory vs. hospitalized status had little effect on nurses' judgments about extent of suffering. The highly significant difference in response to the illness variable appears to be a function of the amount of visible pathology.

The initial hypotheses that posited relationships between the degree of suffering inferred and similarity of patient and nurse in age or social class were not supported. No relationship was found to support a hypothesis that response to patients' verbalizations would differ as a result of nurse-patient similarity. (See Figures 1 and 2.)

Subjects' rankings of the relative usefulness of eleven cues in assessing suffering are shown in Table III. Neither subject age nor social class markedly influenced the ratings. The two most important factors were facial expression and diagnosis. The relative ranking of requests for relief and verbalization of distress was consistent with subjects' responses to these cues in

TABLE II

Mean Inferred Suffering Scores, Standard Deviations, and F Scores for Patients with Various Characteristics

Patient Characteristic	Mean Score	Standard Deviation	F Score	Significance Level
Age				
Young	3.0507	.55		
Middle age	3.0794	.54		
Older	3.1576	.55		
			22.599	$p < .0005$
Social Class				
High	3.1169	.54		
Middle	3.0703	.53		
Low	3.1019	.55		
			6.379	$p < .005$
Verbalization				
Verbal	3.2236	.57		
Nonverbal	2.9690	.54		
			112.335	$p < .0005$
Statement Type				
Complaint	3.1770	.60		
Request	3.2500	.62		
			6.162	$p < .025$
Diagnosis				
Leg abscess	3.4077	.59		
Hematoma of finger	3.2049	.78		
Otitis media	2.7765	.87		
Pneumonia	2.8015	.64		
Polypectomy	3.4938	.61		
Phlebitis	2.8947	.56		
			69.177	$p < .0005$
Sex				
Female	3.0914	.53		
Male	3.1013	.54		
			1.276	N.S.

TABLE III

Mean Rating and Rank Value Assigned to Eleven Factors in
Order of Usefulness to Nurse in Assessing Degree of Suffering

Patient Factor	Mean Rating	Rank
Facial Expression	3.102	1
Diagnosis	3.142	2
Position and Movements	3.884	3
Vocalization	4.605	4
Request for Relief	5.225	5
Verbalization	5.694	6
Age	6.463	7
Prognosis	6.612	8
Ethnicity	8.469	9
Sex	8.952	10
Social Class	9.714	11

the vignettes. The avowed unimportance of social class as a
cue is at variance with the actual use of this cue.

Content analysis of the subjects' written definitions of suffering suggested that nurses cannot readily organize their empirical evidence into coherent operational definitions. While
22 per cent defined suffering as wholly physical, the majority
said that suffering involves feelings of physical and/or emotional discomfort or distress in response to a variety of physical
and/or psychological stimuli. No association was noted between differences in suggested cause or differences in description of phenomena associated with suffering, in the subjects'
definitions, and the degrees of suffering they inferred from the
vignettes.

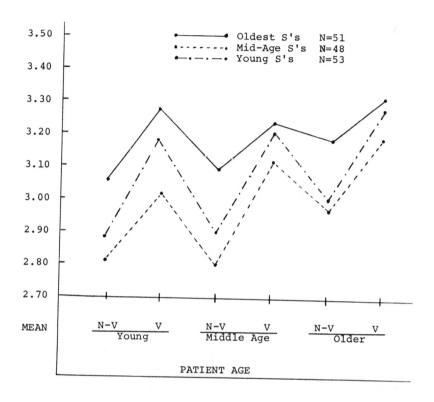

FIGURE 1

Mean Degree of Suffering Inferred by Three Nurse Age
Groups for Verbal and Non-Verbal Patients in Three Age
Groups

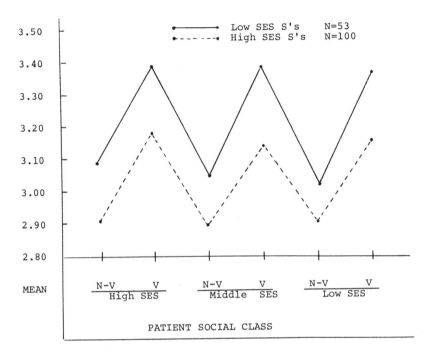

FIGURE 2

Mean Degree of Suffering Inferred by High and Low SES
Nurses for Verbal and Non-Verbal Patients in Three Social
Classes

DISCUSSION AND IMPLICATIONS

Comparison of the findings of this study with those reported by Davitz and her associates (Davitz & Pendleton, 1969)
reveals a number of differences regarding the relationship of
the age and social class of patients and the degree to which
they are believed by nurses to be suffering. Davitz and Pendleton reported that young adults were rated as suffering significantly more than aged patients, while in the current study the
subjects inferred the greatest suffering among the oldest
patients described and the least for the middle-aged and
youngest groups. These findings appear contradictory until

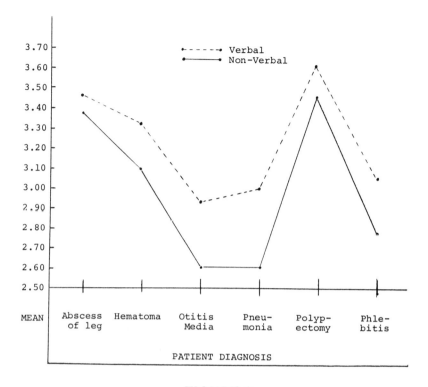

FIGURE 3

Comparison of Mean Degree of Suffering Inferred by Nurses
for Verbal and Non-Verbal Patients by Patient Diagnosis.

placed in the perspective of the degree of illness described in
the two studies. The situations used in the Davitz instrument
involved only critically ill patients, some of whom had a poor
prognosis, whereas the patients described in the current study
were, at the most, moderately ill. While both studies support a
general hypothesis that the degree of suffering inferred is related to the age of the patient, the combined results strongly
suggest an interaction of patient age and acuity of illness that
differentially affects the degree to which a given patient is believed to suffer. Testing of such a hypothesis, using a wider
range of illness categories, would seem a fruitful line for
further inquiry.

The findings from both the present and the prior study also support a general hypothesis that the degree of suffering inferred by the nurse is related to the social class of the patient. As was the case with the age variable, however, some discrepancies between the two sets of data must be noted. Davitz found that the degree of suffering inferred for upper class patients was significantly less than that inferred for the middle and lower classes, but a complete reversal of this relationship emerges from the present data. We might suspect, as in the case of patient age, some interaction of social class and acuity of illness. A more likely possibility might be that the nurse, from an essentially middle class point of view, expects the middle class patient to "bear up" in the face of mild to moderate disease but becomes increasingly sympathetic as the acuity of disease increases for such individuals. Thus, the hypothesized relationship between social class similarity of nurse and patient and the degree of suffering inferred by the nurse might be supported if widely ranging disease conditions were considered as intervening variables.

Interestingly, although the subjects stated in the rank-order question that the patients' social class was an unimportant factor in their judgments of suffering, social class did have an effect on the ratings. The overt denial of the usefulness of this cue may illustrate an ideological conflict between the norm of patient equality and the norm of individualization. Faced with the exigency of multiple situations presented for their judgment, the subjects did in fact utilize the social class cue. When later required to attach a relative value to this factor, they denied its importance, apparently reverting to espousal of the more normative ideal of social equality.

The predicted relationship between the nurse's self-perceived social class and the amount of suffering inferred was supported by the data, with low SES subjects consistently inferring more suffering than high SES subjects. The literature suggests that lower class individuals have lower pain thresholds and that complaints of physical pain may be used by this group to signify other suffering. Further, they are under less social constraint to minimize their suffering and in most situations are free to share their difficulties with others. The lower class nurse, to the extent that she shares these attitudes and responses toward suffering, apparently tends not to minimize the suffering of others. The upper class nurses, on the other hand, may be under social constraint to minimize their own suffering; the results suggest that they extend this norm to their expectations of others as well.

Failure to demonstrate a significant relationship between the age of the nurse and the degree of suffering inferred was in some ways surprising. Intuitively, one might expect some age-correlated changes either as a function of repeated exposure to the suffering of others over time or as the result of wider life experiences generally. One possible explanation of the failure to demonstrate an age relationship, if one in fact exists, may be methodological. The total age range of subjects was determined by the age of the working population. There were no gaps between age groups and, in effect, the groups may have represented a continuum. Replication with more sharply defined age groupings would seem indicated.

Whether or not the patient made a statement indicating that he believed himself to be suffering had a marked and highly significant effect on the degree of suffering the subjects inferred. This finding seems to indicate that the patients' statements were believed; the individual who complained of distress was assumed to be suffering more than similar individuals who did not complain. This is consistent with other findings about the importance of the patient's verbalization as a cue for the nurse.

A difference in nurse response was also noted in relation to the type of statement made by the patient. Patients who made a direct request for medication or other relief measures were invariably rated as suffering more than those who simply verbalized distress without a specific request. On the surface, this suggests that a request for relief is taken somewhat more seriously by the nurse, a supposition supported by the relative ranking subjects gave to these two cues. The possibility of methodological artifact must also be considered. In the clinical setting the nurse has the opportunity to verify most cues by seeking additional information, a condition not available to the study subjects.

The literature does suggest that pain must be fairly severe before patients are willing to request relief. On the other hand, the generalized complaints of distress may have seemed equivocal, in that subjects could not ask the patient who said "I feel so terrible" exactly what he meant by that statement; such verbalizations may then have conveyed less information about the actual state of the patient. An investigation of the relative cue value of various types of distress statements might serve to clarify the present findings.

Because of the relative paucity of cues given in the patient descriptions, subject response to each of these factors may have been somewhat inflated. That is, some of the cues may be quite unimportant when they occur in less isolated form in the clinical setting. Particular caution must be exercised in relation to conclusions about the subjects' response to patient statements of distress. In the rank-order question, factors relating to how the patient actually looks were rated as more important than either statements of distress or requests for relief. Verbal behavior can be contradicted by nonverbal behavior, and people are more likely to trust and believe a nonverbal message than a verbal one when the two are contradictory (Knapp, 1972, p. 9). The significance to the nurse of a particular verbal statement may depend as much on how it is said as on the actual content of the message; the circumstances may, in fact, convey more information than the verbal message. Further study is recommended to determine which patient behaviors might be associated with the nurse's acceptance or rejection of a statement of distress.

The mean scores for the various diseases might be considered to be the baseline level of suffering the subjects expected to encounter with each condition, in all probability based on prior experience with similar illnesses. Strauss and his associates have noted that such pre-existing standards remain salient as long as the patient exhibits behavior consistent with the expectation (Strauss, Fagerhaugh, & Glaser, 1974). There was a fairly constant mean increase from nonverbal to verbal items in the four categories with highest baseline scores. The very marked increase in response to verbal patients with diseases for which relatively little suffering is expected (pneumonia and otitis media) seems to suggest that the study subjects had no difficulty in revising their estimates upward in the face of additional evidence of suffering. (See Figure 3.) The literature does suggest that patient behaviors and complaints that are not consistent with the nurse's expectation tend to be disregarded, in which case we might have expected little change in the face of a distress signal from patients whose baseline score was low.

The marked main effect of diagnosis on the ratings of suffering was not surprising, given the instrumentation employed for the study. Since age and occupation alone can give little, if any, indication of the presence or absence of suffering, the diagnostic information was the major viable cue in half of the items. That the subjects were able, given such items, to formulate judgments that were quite well differentiated on the basis of diagnosis, supports the suggestions found in the literature regarding expected trajectories associated with various conditions. It is important to note, in this connection, that patients' self-perception of their own distress has been found to bear no relationship to their diagnosis. Patients make judgments about how they feel, while nurses appear to judge how they think the patient *should* feel under the circumstances.

The finding that the degree of suffering inferred was related to the amount of visible pathology associated with various disease conditions strongly suggests that the subjects were using an acute pain model, rather than a more generalized model of suffering, as the basis for their judgments. This supposition is further supported by the subjects' ranking of the importance of various cues. The patient's facial expression, his position and body movements, and such vocalizations as crying or moaning were all accorded considerable importance as cues. Thus it appears that, in addition to the visibility of pathology, high visibility of patient response to suffering is also essential.

The patient's prognosis might be assumed to be closely related to diagnosis in cue value if a general model of suffering was conceptualized by the subjects. In the rank-order question, however, subjects considered diagnosis as very important in the judgment process but accorded little importance to prognosis. Again, this suggests the subjects we·e thinking of acute pain associated with immediate circumstances rather than using a broader concept of suffering including other than pain responses.

The conceptual framework for this study suggested that nurse-patient similarity would have a differential effect on the degree of suffering inferred by the nurse. None of the hypotheses relating to similarity was supported by the data. The question that arises at this juncture is whether or not any of the similarity hypotheses were, in fact, tested in this study. While we can assume that certain similarities existed between the subjects and the patients described, there is no way of determining whether these similarities were actually perceived as such by the study subjects. Particularly tenuous in this regard is the assumed similarity on the basis of social class since the patient's occupation (and by extension, income) was the sole social class indicator given. Quite possibly, any real feeling of similarity with another would require some interpersonal communication to determine common interests and ideals. Certainly the written descriptions could give little clue to the patient's personality or attitudes, factors that might be important in formulating feelings of similarity in the absence of other knowledge. The failure to support the similarity hypothesis may, then, be due to a weakness in the study design.

Any discussion of the findings relating to the subjects' written definitions of suffering must be prefaced by examination of the limitations of the methodology employed. The task faced by the subjects was not a simple one, considering the difficulties philosophers and scientists have experienced in attempting to define pain and suffering: clear and precise definitions of abstract concepts are not quickly conceived. In addition, even when a problem seems fairly clear, individuals may have considerable difficulty in finding terms that precisely convey their intended meaning. Most of the subjects did focus their thoughts sufficiently to deal with an identification of the nature of the phenomena associated with suffering. The ideas that subjects presented beyond the basic description of phenomena were quite varied, and in many cases somewhat disorganized and unfocused; they must therefore be treated as suggestive, rather than conclusive, evidence of how nurses define suffering.

The findings relating to the nature of the phenomena produced by suffering strongly suggest that most nurses hold a rather broad definition that includes both emotional and physical distress, although over 22 per cent of the respondents discussed the sufferer's symptoms as being solely physical.

An interesting finding was that the high social class subjects, with somewhat greater frequency than the low self-raters, tended to talk about suffering in terms of physical causes and physical effects. While no statistical difference was found between the mean suffering scores of subjects giving the two different causal definitions, the lower class subjects did have significantly higher mean scores than the upper class subjects. This suggests that a relationship between definition of and inferences about suffering may, in fact, exist. Further, it suggests that when suffering is defined as both physical and emotional, the total effect is seen as additive and results in inferences of greater suffering.

Some subjects attempted to give operational definitions of the concept by discussing various cues they look for in order to determine the amount of suffering being experienced. In view of the frequency with which nurses are called upon to make judgments about the distress of others, it is perhaps surprising that more of the subjects did not take this approach. As in the rank-order question, the observed intensity of distress was emphasized by the subjects. This raises serious questions about nurse response to individuals who are not particularly demonstrative, or who do not exhibit overt signs of distress. Is the distress of a chronically ill individual likely to go unheeded because he doesn't look particularly uncomfortable?

If indeed the nurses accepted the currently voguish definition of suffering as "whatever the sufferer says it is" (McCaffery, 1972, p. 8), as their response to the inference items suggests, their written definitions did not reflect it. Rather, it appears that a patient's statement gains validity only when measured against other more important cues.

Perhaps the most striking thing about the subjects' definitions was their general lack of focus and a certain quality of randomness, almost as though a few stray thoughts were garnered and jotted down. Although this may have been a function of the difficulty of the task or of subject fatigue, these nurses had just finished formulating a series of judgments about the degree to which they believed patients to be suffering. If they had any really coherent definitional standard in mind, they seemed unable to state it clearly. It may be that the nurse calls upon now subconscious past observations to reach what appear to be intuitive conclusions about the present circumstance. But if such past observation has never been organized, it is useful only when patient behavior conforms exactly to that previously observed. This provides no framework within which new situations may be measured, and the behavior of the sufferer who deviates from the expected is likely to be misunderstood.

The recent nursing literature has stressed the need for theoretical bases for nursing practice—theories founded in the nature of man in relation to his environment. The process of nursing is primarily one of problem solving, but solutions are sometimes hard come by when the nature of the problem is unknown or ill defined. If nursing care involves the diagnosing of human responses, then we need to know considerably more about these responses, and that knowledge needs to be part of the armamentarium the nurse brings to the practice situation. Recent research has begun to explore the contingencies surrounding the experiences of pain and suffering, and no doubt will continue to add to our knowledge of this complex problem; but as yet, little of this new knowledge has found its way into the practice of nurses.

Had the subjects been required to give definitions of such medical problems as surgical shock or insulin reaction, they would have had little difficulty stating cause and effect, or delineating the signs and symptoms they would look for. But when faced with the necessity of defining the concept of suffering, a nursing care problem, they found themselves at a loss for words. While there can be little question about the complexity of that problem we have called suffering, it is more than a little disturbing to find that practitioners who deal with suffering daily apparently lack the knowledge base from which to do so.

The nucleus of such a knowledge base, considering the centrality of suffering as a nursing care problem, should form an important portion of the basic education of nurses. Part of our failure to give students a good grounding in this area may be attributable to a lack of nursing theory pertaining to suffering as a human response, and to a failure, until recently, to pull together and organize those facts and theories that are available. Certainly most nurses beginning in practice believe that the relief of suffering is a major nursing function and have every intention of fulfilling this function. Good intentions, however, are rarely sufficient. Our recognition of suffering needs to go beyond the intuitive; nurses need a basis in fact in order to identify and respond to patient needs.

One major implication of this study for nurses who must regularly evaluate the suffering of others lies in the extent to which the practitioner's characteristics and personality may enter into the process. Although only one factor, the self-perceived social status of the nurse, was shown in this study to be related, there are undoubtedly others equally or more important. It is unlikely that the subjects were aware of the extent to which this single variable influenced what they said about patients; probably they would have denied such an effect had they been asked. Nurses are admonished to bring all available resources to bear when they approach patient care problems, yet how often do they rely upon understanding of that resource which is always available to them—their own selves, unique and individual?

The individuality of patients is frequently stressed; individual differences are part of the human condition. Paradoxically, the individuality of any particular nurse tends to become submerged in a kind of generic being called "the nurse," with an underlying assumption that one nurse is much like the next. A scientific and factual base must be coupled with sensitivity to another's state—a sensitivity that might be characterized as the *art* of nursing. It is here that the nurse's individual characteristics and talents become a major resource. If this resource is to be used in a purposeful way, undergraduate programs will have to foster self-knowledge. Further, faculties will have to teach alternative nursing care approaches that consider not only the patient as an individual, but the nurse as an individual as well.

Empathy, the sharing and understanding of another's state of mind, is more likely to arise between individuals who share important characteristics. Similarity and empathy may both, then, be related not only to what appears at times to be an intuitive apprehension of another's distress but also to the extent to which the nurse's evaluation matches the patient's own evaluation of his state. There is a need to increase nurse awareness of the possibility of, and reasons for, their failure to fully understand (or even like) some patients, with a concomitant awareness that such failures may be largely circumstantial. This might do much to reduce guilt feelings engendered by inability to solve particular problems, and thus might encourage consultation with others and make possible withdrawal from unproductive relationships.

All nursing, whether it focuses on well or ill individuals, is in a very broad sense intended to relieve or prevent suffering. In the last analysis, we must perhaps acknowledge that our knowledge base for understanding and identifying suffering is scant, and in some respects inaccurate, and that our knowledge of the cognitive processes involved in making clinical judgments is less than complete. Expansion of the knowledge base in both these areas is essential if nurses are to be taught to perform this basic role successfully.

REFERENCES

Baer, Eva; Davitz, Lois J.; Lieb, Renee. "Inferences of Physical Pain and Psychological Distress in Relation to Verbal and Nonverbal Patient Communication." *Nursing Research* 19 (1970):388–391.

Baron, Robert A. "Magnitude of Model's Apparent Pain and Ability to Aid the Model as Determinants of Observer Reaction Time." *Psychonomic Science* 21 (1970):196–197.

Blaylock, Jerry Naomi. "Characteristics of Nurses and of Medical-Surgical Patients to Whom They React Positively and Negatively." Ed.D. dissertation, Teachers College, Columbia University, 1970.

Brown, Roger. *Social Psychology*. New York: Free Press, 1965.

Copp, Laurel A. "The Spectrum of Suffering." *American Journal of Nursing* 74 (1974):491–495.

Davitz, Lois J. & Pendleton, Sydney H. "Nurses' Inferences of Suffering." *Nursing Research* 18 (1969):100–107.

Ekdawi, M.Y. "The Difficult Patient." *British Journal of Psychiatry* 113 (1967):547–552.

Glaser, Barney G., & Strauss, Anselm L. *Awareness of Dying*. Chicago: Aldine, 1965.

——— *Time for Dying*. Chicago: Aldine, 1968.

Gonda, Thomas A. "Some Remarks on Pain." *Bulletin, British Psychological Society* 47 (April 1962):29–35.

Graffam, Shirley R. "Nurse Response to the Patient in Distress." *Nursing Research* 19 (1970):331–336.

Hackett, Thomas P. "Pain and Prejudice: Why Do We Doubt that the Patient Is in Pain?" *Medical Times* 99 (1971):130–141.

Hammond, Kenneth R. "Clinical Inference in Nursing: A Psychologist's Viewpoint." *Nursing Research* 15 (1966):27–38.

Hammond, Kenneth R., et al. "Clinical Inference in Nursing: Analyzing Cognitive Tasks Representative of Nursing Problems." *Nursing Research* 15 (1966):134–138.(a)

———. "Clinical Inference in Nursing: Information Units Used. *Nursing Research* 15 (1966):236–243.(b)

———."Clinical Inference in Nursing: Use of Information-Seeking Strategies by Nurses." *Nursing Research* 15 (1966):330–336.(c)

———. "Clinical Inference in Nursing: Revising Judgments." *Nursing Research* 16 (1967):38–45.

Hornstein, Harvey A. "Promotive Tension: The Basis of Prosocial Behavior from a Lewinian Perspective." *Journal of Social Issues* 28 (1972):191–218.

Jacox, Ada, & Stewart, Mary. *Psychosocial Contingencies of the Pain Experience*. Iowa City: Univ. of Iowa, 1973.

Kelly, Katherine J. "An Approach to the Study of Clinical Inference in Nursing: Introduction." *Nursing Research* 13 (1964):314–315.(a)

———"Utilization of the 'Lens Model' Method to Study the Inferential Process of the Nurse." *Nursing Research* 13 (1964):319–322.(b)

King, Stanley H. *Perceptions of Illness and Medical Practice*. New York: Russell Sage Foundation, 1962.

Knapp, Mark L. *Nonverbal Communication in Human Interaction*. New York: Holt, Rinehart & Winston, 1972.

Lenburg, Carrie B.; Burnside, Helen; & Davitz, Lois J. "Inferences of Physical Pain and Psychological Distress in Relation to Length of Time in the Nursing Education Program." *Nursing Research* 19(1970):399–401.

Lenburg, Carrie B.; Glass, Helen P.; & Davitz, Lois J. "Inferences of Physical Pain and Psychological Distress in Relation to the Stage of the Patient's Illness and Occupation of the Perceiver." *Nursing Research* 19 (1970):392–398.

Lerner, Melvin J., & Simmons, Carolyn H. "Observer's Reaction to the 'Innocent Victim': Compassion or Rejection?" *Journal of Personality and Social Psychology* 4 (1966):203–210.

Lynn, R., & Eysenck, H.J. "Tolerance for Pain, Extraversion and Neuroticism." *Perceptual and Motor Skills* 12 (1961):161–162.

McCaffery, Margo. *Nursing Management of the Patient with Pain*. Philadelphia: J. B. Lippincott, 1972.

Petrie, Asenath. *Individuality in Pain and Suffering*. Chicago: Univ. of Chicago Press, 1967.

Segal, Bernard E. "Nurses and Patients: A Case Study in Stratification." *Journal of Health and Human Behavior* 5 (1964):54–60.

Strauss, Anselm; Fagerhaugh, Y.; & Glaser, Barney. "Pain: An Organizational-Work-Interactional Perspective." *Nursing Outlook* 22 (1974):560–566.

Szasz, Thomas S. *Pain and Pleasure: A Study of Bodily Feelings*. New York: Basic Books, 1957.

——. "Language and Pain." In *American Handbook of Psychiatry* Vol. 1. Edited by S. Arieti. New York: Basic Books, 1959.

Weiss, James M. A., ed. *Nurses, Patients and Social Systems*. Columbia, Mo.: Univ. of Missouri Press, 1968.

Yakimovich, Dorothy, & Saltz, Eli. "Helping Behavior." *Psychonomic Science* 23 (1971):427–428.

Zborowski, Mark. "Cultural Components in Response to Pain." *Journal of Social Issues* 8 (1952):16–30.

——. *People in Pain*. San Francisco: Jossey-Bass, 1969.

Critique

Sydney H. Pendleton

DR. OBERST IS to be commended for having chosen a topic which is not only interesting and relevant to nursing practice but also because of the subjective nature of suffering, difficult to study. Since the alleviation of suffering is an important part of the work of the nurse, studies of nurses' inferences of suffering may have an impact on the quality of nursing practice.

The author hypothesized that nurse–patient similarity would affect the degree of suffering inferred by the nurse, but she concluded that her data did not support this hypothesis. It may be that she did not compare similar groups of nurses and patients. I have chosen to discuss three areas of nurse–patient similarity, two chosen by the author and one she did not include in her study.

Turning to Dr. Oberst's dissertation (Teachers College, Columbia University, 1975), upon which her paper was based, one finds that the groupings by age and socioeconomic status were dissimilar for the nurses and the patients. The nurses were divided into three groups by age: 20–29, 30–44, and over 45. The oldest nurse was 65. The patients described in the written items were also divided into three groups by age: 17–25, 35–50, and 65 and over. It is immediately apparent that there is little nurse–patient similarity in these age groupings.

None of the nurses in the study are similar in age to the youngest or oldest patients in the vignettes. This is not surprising. However, if the patients had been grouped so as to correspond to the age groups of the nurses, a better measure of similarity might have been obtained. One could have included an under-20 group of patients and an over-65 group of patients in addition to three groups corresponding to the three age groups of the nurses. As it is, the similar and dissimilar are lumped together, which may account for the fact that the author found no significant interaction between the age of the nurse and the age of the patient.

The author found that nurses inferred the greatest amount of suffering in the oldest group of patients. This age group does not correspond to any of the age groups of the nurses. It is possible therefore that nurses infer the least suffering in patients most like themselves.

The second area of nurse–patient similarity considered was socioeconomic status. The socioeconomic status of the patients was classified as high, middle, or low. Using Hamburger's classification, the author determined the socioeconomic status of the patients according to their occupations or those of their spouses.

The question of how to define the socioeconomic status of working women is not an easy one. Traditionally the socioeconomic status of a woman has depended upon the status of the male upon whom she is dependent: her father or her husband. The working woman, however, could be classified *either* on the basis of her own profession, education, and income *or* on the basis of the status of her husband or father. The fact that the subjects rated themselves does not eliminate this factor. Does the nurse, wife of a dentist, rate herself the same as the wife of a dentist in one of the vignettes where the wife's occupation, if any, is not given?

The nurse-subjects rated their own socioeconomic status and, as might have been expected, the ratings clustered around the middle of the six-point scale. However, the author states in her dissertation (p.72) that "because of skewed distribution, the subjects' self-ratings of current SES were compressed into two categories." The nurses, most of whom rated themselves middle class, were artificially divided into high and low socioeconomic status groups.

It is doubtful whether this division into "high" and "low" is meaningful. The nurse-subjects were most similar to the middle class patients in whom they inferred the least pain. The analysis of variance relative to this datum (effect of patients' social class on nurses' inferences of suffering) was significant at the .005 level (as shown in Table II).

Although Dr. Oberst states that none of the three hypotheses relating to similarity were supported by the data, this negative finding may have resulted from the way in which the author divided her subjects into groups. It appears that, given a different treatment of the nurses' social class self-ratings, the author's hypothesis that "The degree of suffering inferred by nurses is related to similarity of the nurses' self-perceived social class and the social class of the patient" (the dissertation, p. 16) *is* supported by the data.

I turn now to another kind of nurse–patient similarity, which is not included in Dr. Oberst's study. The author *has* stressed the importance of certain individual characteristics and talents of nurses, prefacing her discussion with the following comment:

> The individuality of patients is frequently stressed; individual differences are part of the human condition. Paradoxically, the individuality of any particular nurse tends to become submerged in a kind of generic called "the nurse," with an underlying assumption that one nurse is much like the next.

However, she gives us no data on the racial, cultural, or ethnic backgrounds of the nurses who were her subjects. Since previous research has shown that the ethnic or cultural background of the nurse is significant in her inference of suffering, such data would have been quite useful in the present study.

In the case of the patients, the author states in her dissertation (p.61) that "Each patient described was given a name in order to impart as much individuality as possible; the names used were selected to avoid ethnic identification." The following is a sample of the names used: Helen Black, Allison Barber, Hank Sawyer, William Crawford, Teresa Steele. It is not possible to avoid ethnic identification by using Anglo-Saxon names. From these names one could infer that the patients might be black or white but not oriental. They are also not Polish, Italian, or Spanish, for example. How does the Polish or Chinese or Jamaican nurse react to a patient with an Anglo-Saxon name?

Another factor that cannot be eliminated is the influence of the racial and cultural background of the researcher. We each have a frame of reference based on our individual pasts, including our racial and cultural background, which must be taken into account. In addition the researcher must be aware that her racial or ethnic background has an influence on her subjects. This becomes especially important in connection with the type of instrument used in this study. What will the nurse-subjects infer about patients described in a research instrument administered by a researcher of a particular racial and ethnic background?

In the short time available it was not possible to discuss all the areas of Dr. Oberst's study. Therefore I refer you to her dissertation, where these are discussed in detail. Also, the review of the literature there is extensive and most interesting.

Clinical inference is an important part of the nursing process. More studies are needed to identify the cues used in clinical inference and other factors that influence the process. The development of nursing theory in this area would be a significant contribution to the field.

Patients' Definitions of Recovery from Acute Illness

Rose Ann Naughton & Doreen Kolditz

INTRODUCTION

OUR INTEREST in the topic of recovery initially developed as a result of observing patients who were about to be discharged from the hospital. Most patients accepted the physician's decision that they were ready to go home and did so as planned. However, there were two groups of patients who did not leave the hospital as scheduled.

Patients in the first group very directly told the physician that they did not feel ready to go. Their reasons usually had to do with feeling physically unable to leave or with temporary conditions at home. Discharge scheduling was therefore delayed.

In the second group of patients, discharge was scheduled but subsequently delayed by some intervening event, such as an exacerbation of symptomatology, an accident, or the development of new symptoms. This sequence of events took place with enough frequency to raise the question as to whether the event delaying discharge took place because the patient himself did not feel ready to leave the hospital.

These observations prompted the wish to explore the concept of recovery from the patient's point of view. They raised in the minds of the investigators questions like: What is recovery? How do hospitalized patients determine that they have recovered sufficiently from an illness to leave the hospital? How do patients determine that they have recovered fully from an illness? Do patients with varied backgrounds define recovery differently?

A review of the literature uncovered very little about the notion of recovery, particularly as viewed by the patient. There was a great deal, however, on definitions of health and illness, the sick role, and illness behavior. The works of Koos (1954), Saunders (1954), Parsons (1972), and Mechanic (1968) in these areas are widely familiar, as is Zborowski's (1969) study of cultural differences and pain response.

Common to these and other studies was the fact that the sociological variables that characterize groups strongly influence health and illness behavior. Those found to be most influential were socioeconomic status, education, occupation, religion, ethnicity, marital status, sex, and age. The research question of this study evolved accordingly, to become: "What is the relationship between selected sociological variables and patients' definitions of recovery from acute illness?"

THE STUDY

Design: The study undertaken to answer this question was a descriptive one using a survey design. It was exploratory in nature. A rating scale that contained recovery factors was developed. Shortly before they were to be discharged, patients were asked to judge the relative importance of the scale items in determining their recovery. In addition, sociological factors were learned through patient interviews. The influence of the sociological variables on the rating scale responses was then studied.

Since recovery from the patient's point of view had not previously been defined in the literature, it was determined that a baseline definition of this construct should be studied in this research. In delineating a population for study it was decided that a group of patients in which the illness situation was time-limited and institutionally controlled, and in which the fewest number of variables existed concerning the illness, would be desirable. Therefore, it was decided that patients who were essentially "well" before hospitalization, who required abdominal surgery for a benign condition, who then recovered without complications, and who would be expected to return to their usual level of functioning, could provide this baseline definition of recovery. Acute illness was thus operationally defined.

The Instrument: The categories of the instrument used in the study were developed primarily through a series of open-ended questions concerning perceptions of recovery; the questions were asked of hospitalized patients who had recently had surgery.

It was learned immediately that patients are very present-oriented in the early post-operative phase of recovery. Many who had IV's or tubes, or were NPO or bedridden, reported that they would be recovered when they could eat and/or walk again and when the IV's and tubes were removed. It was learned further that patients distinguished very sharply between factors indicating readiness to leave the hospital and those indicating full recovery.

Since our interest was to determine the patient's definitions of these two later phases of recovery (*readiness for discharge* from the hospital and subsequent *full recovery*), it was decided to interview patients who had already negotiated the immediate post-operative phase and whose discharge was imminent. The patients interviewed were thus all ambulatory, on oral feedings, and without IV's or tubes in place.

As seen in Tables 1 and 2, information gleaned from patients in relation both to readiness for discharge and to full recovery constituted two major kinds of *cues to recovery:* internal cues, which the patient felt and could monitor; and external cues, which came from people or events in the environment.

Internal cues were in three major categories: physical, feeling tone, and capability. The *physical* cues dealt with the direct sequellae of the surgery: the status of the wound and the resultant pain. They referred also to strength and energy level, and to return of appetite and sleep patterns. *Feeling tone* cues dealt with emotional responses to the surgical event, such as fear, worry, and level of "spirits." *Capability* cues concerned the ability to resume self-care and mobility and activities at home.

External cues to recovery emanated from medical and nursing staff and from the patient's family and friends. Cues from the professional staff consisted of the actual discharge decision and staff activities that indicated improvement in the patient's condition. Cues from family and friends were essentially their expressed opinions of the patient's health status and behaviors indicating that they felt the patient was recovering and could resume his usual role and responsibilities.

The format of the instrument was a rating scale. During the field trials of the instrument it was learned that the most efficient way to determine the relative weight of the several cues to recovery was to ask the patient to rate each cue as "very important," "somewhat important," or "not important" in determining recovery. Each patient responded to both parts of the scale: first to the 25 Readiness for Discharge cues, then to the 12 for Full Recovery. Those items rated "very important" by the majority of patients were considered the major components of a definition of recovery for patients similar to those in this study.

The patient was also asked which of all the cues was "most important" and who was the "best judge" of his recovery. Finally, patients were asked to estimate the length of time it would take for them to be fully recovered.

The Sample: The sample consisted of 200 subjects—99 females and 101 males—who ranged in age from 20 to 70 years. The majority of patients were married, and most were born in the United States. Ethnic group representation was 64% White, 25% Black and 10% Hispanic. The major religious groupings were quite evenly represented. All subjects were ambulatory, eating solid foods, and considered ready for discharge within one to five days.

The Hollingshead Two Factor Index of Social Position (education and occupation being the two factors) was used to determine the socioeconomic status of the subjects. Except for the lowest educational category, there was substantial representation in all groupings.

Most patients were five to seven days post-surgery. Forty-nine percent had herniorrhaphies and the remainder major abdominal surgery. Since the herniorrhaphy does not involve as extensive surgery and anesthesia time as the other procedures, and as a result the recovery time is smoother and swifter, data for the two groups were analyzed separately.

Institutions: Data were collected at four large medical centers in the New York area. Three of the hospitals were located in the metropolitan area. One of the institutions was located

TABLE 1

Cue Categories in Readiness for Discharge Scale

INTERNAL CUES

Physical Cues

My wound is healed or almost healed.
My appetite is getting back to normal.
I have no pain or only slight pain.
I'm getting stronger and my energy is increasing.
My sleeping is getting back to normal.

Feeling Tone Cues

My spirits are getting back to normal.
I feel less afraid.
I feel less worried about being sick.
I feel less down in the dumps.
I feel ready to go home.

Capability Cues

I am able to get around without help.
I am able to go outside without help.
I can do things for myself, for instance, wash, walk, dress.
I have no worries how I'll manage at home.
I'll be able to do light work around the house, shopping, cooking, etc.

EXTERNAL CUES

Cues from Medical and Nursing Personnel

My blood pressure and temperature are taken less.
I get fewer medicines.
The doctor tells me I'm ready to go home.
The nurses tell me I'm ready to do more for myself.
The doctors and nurses come to see me less often.

Cues from Family and Friends

My friends and family tell me I'm looking better.
My friends and family tell me I'm ready to go home.
My family and friends don't worry about me like they did after the operation.
Others tell me about the problems at home.
My family and friends treat me more as usual.

TABLE 2

Cue Categories in Full Recovery Scale

INTERNAL CUES

Physical Cues

My pain has disappeared.
My wound is healed.
My sleeping is back to normal.
My appetite is back to normal.
My energy is back to normal.

Feeling Tone Cues

My spirits are back to normal.
I no longer worry about problems with my operation.
I feel fully recovered.

Capability Cues

I'm able to carry out my usual activities, like using public transportation, going to work, driving, shopping, sports, going to meetings, etc.
I'm able to carry out my usual activities, like housework, repairs around the house, hobbies, etc.

EXTERNAL CUES

My doctor says I'm fully recovered.
My family allows me to take on my usual responsibilities.

near the city line but served a predominantly suburban popu-lation. All of the hospitals with the exception of the municipal hospital had private, semi-private, and service patients. Of the three voluntary hospitals, only one permitted the participation of private patients in the study.

Data Collection Procedures: The sample may be described as a convenience sample. Each of the two investigators col-lected data at all hospitals and continued until each had in-terviewed a total of 100 subjects. Originally, it had been our intent to include in the study every patient at all four hospitals who met the selection criteria until the 200 subject quota was reached. However, it soon became apparent that this was not possible. Patients were admitted and discharged with such ir-regularity that it was impossible to be present in the hospitals at the times required by the study criteria. Therefore, all four hospitals were visited twice a week on days that provided the most patients for interview (depending on operative routines and schedules). Following this procedure, the data collection required nine months.

Limitations: There are many limitations in this study refer-rable to its design, the size and sample composition, and the applicability of results. The investigators wish to acknowledge these and others. In particular, the concentration in the data analysis was on sociological variables. Responses are also in-fluenced by other factors, including psychological variables, which were not considered.

Data Analysis: The results of the study consist of three types of data: (1) a frequency distribution of responses to all items on the rating scale; (2) significance levels based on Chi-square values obtained as the result of a bivariate cross-tabulation of demographic characteristics and responses in the rating sheet; and (3) significance levels using Chi-square values that resulted from a multivariate cross-tabulation. Here, the relationship be-tween two variables was stratified according to the categories of a test factor to determine whether or not the two-variable relationship was real or influenced by the third variable (Ro-senberg, 1968, p. 201).

RESULTS AND INTERPRETATIONS

In interpreting the study results two facts should be kept in mind. First, primary emphasis in the data analysis was placed on the percentage of subjects who chose an item as "very important" on the rating scale. Each patient had to make a distinct choice in selecting a level of importance for an item, thereby rejecting two other levels. Compiling the results on those items chosen as "very important" should provide an outline of the most salient components of a definition of recovery for patients similar to those in this study. Second, in relation to the rank order procedure used in this study, subjects were not asked to rank the factors in order of importance; rather, the investigators placed the factors into ranks based on the percentage of "very important" responses received.

In presenting the results, first the frequency distributions of responses to the recovery factors will be discussed, and then the influence of the sociological variables on responses will be presented.

DEFINITIONS OF RECOVERY: *Readiness for Discharge*

If health professionals were polled as to the factors most important in determining a surgical patient's readiness for discharge, they would more than likely cite the state of the patient's wound, his temperature, and other physical factors directly related to the surgery. Patients see it differently.

As seen in Table 3, more than 57% of all subjects regarded the items in the first eleven ranks as "very important" in determining their readiness to leave the hospital. The concerns expressed in these items may be seen as representing the major components of the patient's definition of a level of recovery sufficient to leave the hospital. They may be grouped as four   components:

1. The patient's estimation of his energy and capabilities.
2. The patient's feeling state.
3. The healing of the wound and level of pain.
4. The doctor's indication of discharge readiness.

TABLE 3

Rank Order of "Very Important" Responses To Cues
To Readiness For Discharge

RANK	RESPONSE	PERCENT
1	I'm getting stronger and my energy is increasing	88
2	I am able to get around without help.	83.5
3.5	I can do things for myself, for instance, wash, walk, dress, etc.	83
3.5	The doctor tells me I'm ready to go home.	83
5	I feel ready to go home.	82.5
6	My wound is healed or almost healed.	71
7	My spirits are getting back to normal.	70
8	I am able to go outside without help.	65
9	I have no worries about how I'll manage at home.	64
10	I have no pain or only slight pain.	59.5
11	I feel less worried about being sick.	57
12	My appetite is getting back to normal.	48
13.5	My blood pressure and temperature are taken less often.	47.5
13.5	I feel less afraid.	47.5
15	My sleeping is getting back to normal.	46
16	The nurses tell me I'm ready to do more for myself.	45.5
17	I get fewer medicines.	44.5
18	I feel less down in the dumps.	44
19	My friends and family tell me I'm looking better.	43
20	My family and friends treat me more as usual.	41.5
21	The doctors and nurses come to see me less often.	40.5
22	My family and friends don't worry about me like they did after the operation.	39.5
23	I'll be able to do light work around the house; shopping, cooking, etc.	36.5
24	My friends and family tell me I'm ready to go home.	26
25	Others tell me about the problems at home.	16

The selection of "I'm getting stronger . . ." as "very important" by 88% of the patients was very striking and quite unexpected. No matter what the type of operation or the length of time since the operation, patients considered this item "very important." This raised the question as to whether this was purely a physical response to the surgical event, as its placement on the rating scale would indicate.

Surgery of all kinds can deplete strength and energy, but the degree of depletion would seem to depend on the extent of surgery. The patient response here raised a big question in the minds of the investigators as to whether the *emotional response* to surgery of *any type* (and emotional response certainly can have physical manifestations) was a large part of the overwhelming concern for strength and energy levels. The physical trauma involved in different types of surgery varies. Is it possible that the emotional trauma does not vary as greatly? Very much allied to this notion is the fact that three of the first eleven ranked items dealt specifically with emotional responses associated with hospitalization and surgery.

No one would deny the fusion of physical and emotional responses in any situation. We all preach man's wholeness and a holistic approach in dealings with people. But is attention to emotional responses really incorporated in the plans of care for "routine" surgical patients? This research certainly indicates a need for such attention.

In numerous data collection interviews, patients discussed feelings of sadness and dejection after surgery. Several patients described uncontrollable crying episodes, which were brought on by no apparent reason since everything directly connected with the operation was progressing smoothly. One patient described her crying as "post-operative blues" and likened it to her "post-partum blues" of many years before. Recalling previous surgery, some patients told of similar occurrences at the time of discharge or after they had gone home. All of these episodes of dejection were short-lived. Several patients described being frightened by their emotional reactions in this period because they could not understand them.

Several theories might explain the emotional responses referred to by patients. They may be a depressive reaction to the surgical experience, as described by Burgess and Lazare (1973, p.181). Carlson (1970,p.98) describes grief reactions precipitated by loss: the loss of identity respect and individuality in the hospital situation or, as often in the case of surgery, the loss of an organ. The behavior could also be a response to surgery perceived as a crisis, as formulated by Lindemann (1965, p.7), or possibly an emotional letdown response after a period of high tension. Whatever theoretical formulation is used to explain the phenomenon, distressing emotional reactions are a very real part of the surgical experience.

Another major concern of patients is the ability to be independent in daily activities in the hospital and at home. Four of the first eleven ranked items dealt with this. In many instances, the patient in the early post-operative period is unable to carry out daily activities without assistance. This helplessness and dependence is a major indication of the patient's impaired status and necessitates his remaining in the hospital. Independence in these activities was clearly perceived by the patients in this study as a requisite for discharge.

The wound and resultant pain are the direct sequellae of the operative event. As expected, proper healing and pain level were considered very important by large percentages of the patient sample (71% and 59.5% respectively). Many had interesting comments in relation to these two factors. Some said that the wound was the doctor's business and so wasn't their biggest concern in relation to discharge. In relation to pain, a large number indicated that "You have to expect pain with an operation," so that too wasn't considered as important as other criteria of readiness for discharge. It is interesting to note where these two criteria rank in relation to other factors.

Ten of the first eleven ranked items are essentially internal cues to recovery, which the patient can feel and monitor himself. The only external recovery cue that more than 50% of patients regarded as "very important" was "The doctor tells me I'm ready to go home" (83%). Not unexpectedly, the physician's prominence in determining the patient's recovery level was great. Some patients commented that the doctor's opinion was the only important consideration in relation to discharge and recovery.

The importance of the physician's opinion was shown also

in the response to the two open questions at the end of Part I of the rating scale. When asked which of all the items listed was "most important" to the patient in determining his readiness for discharge, the highest proportion, 36% cited the doctor's opinion. (All other responses were scattered.) In addition, the doctor was chosen by 64% of all subjects as the "best judge" of the patient's readiness for discharge.

Items considered "very important" by less than 50% of patients were primarily external cues to recovery. It would appear that the post-operative period is very much one of egocentrism: aside from the physician's opinion, what is most important to the patient are his own feelings and sensations.

In summary then, patients' definitions of a level of recovery that will safely permit them to leave the hospital encompass several themes:

1. Indications of the resolution of the direct sequellae of the surgery.
2. Indications of the resolution of the physical and emotional responses to the surgery.
3. Corroboration by the physician that the patient is well enough to leave the hospital.

DEFINITIONS OF RECOVERY: *Full Recovery*

As seen in Table 4, a large proportion (57–89%) of all patients regarded *all* of the items in the Full Recovery Scale as "very important." Apparently, in order for the patient to consider himself fully recovered, all of the sequellae of the operation must be resolved. Energy, sleep, and appetite must be back to normal. The wound must be healed and pain must have disappeared. The patient must "feel" fully recovered, his spirits must be back to normal, and he must no longer have any worries about the operation. In addition, and perhaps most important, the patient must be able to return to his usual activities and have his family's sanction for this. Finally, the doctor must agree that the patient is fully recovered.

This very positive response to *all* factors of the scale raised several questions. Were these indeed the components of a definition of full recovery, and did this account for the response? Could the response be explained by the fact that there were

TABLE 4

Rank Order of "Very Important" Responses
To Cues to Full Recovery

Rank	Responses	Percent
1	My energy is back to normal	89.5
2	I feel fully recovered	88.5
3	I am able to carry out my usual activities, like using public transportation, going to work, driving, shopping, sports, meetings, etc.	86.5
4	My wound is healed	81.5
5	My pain has disappeared	79.5
6	I'm able to carry out my usual activities, like housework, repairs around the house, hobbies, etc.	76.5
7	My doctor says I'm fully recovered	74
8	I no longer worry about problems with my operation	70
9	My spirits are back to normal	66
10	My family allows me to take on my usual responsibilities	62
11	My sleeping is back to normal	60
12	My appetite is back to normal	57

less than half as many factors on this scale as on the previous scale? Or possibly, since the patient was projecting ahead in time, and not actually in the stage of full recovery, were the responses inflated? Only a similar study conducted perhaps three to six months after discharge could have answered these questions precisely.

A number of the responses concerning full recovery are striking. Again, the notion of energy level, as in the discharge scale, was regarded as very important by the highest proportion of all patients. Strength and energy are obviously depleted to some extent as a result of the operative experience. The question of the specific meaning to patients of the concept of energy again arises. Is this purely a physical phenomenon, or could energy level also be affected by emotional response to the complex of events surrounding hospitalization and surgery? Again: can the physical and emotional effects even be separated?

Parsons (1972, p. 117) defines illness on the basis of inability to carry out the roles and tasks for which the individual has been socialized. The responses of subjects in this study suggest that patients define full recovery from surgery in terms of the ability to resume the activities and responsibilities they were unable to cope with while ill. When the patients were asked which of all the factors was "most important" in determining full recovery, responses were scattered. However, the highest percentage of subjects (32%) chose the ability to resume their usual activities, again emphasizing the value of this capability to patients.

The responses in the full recovery section seem throughout to show great self-reliance on the part of the patient in relation to his recovery. This is in direct contrast to what was seen when patients were defining readiness for discharge. While in the hospital, by virtue of his physical condition, the patient is under the direct supervision of the doctor and the hospital staff. He needs and is dependent on them, and his responses in the discharge scale reflect this. However, as the patient projects himself into his own home and work environment, he tends to view himself more independently and as more responsible for his own well-being. This is shown in the frequency distributions in relation to dependence on the physician's opinion, in the patient's choice of the ability to resume activities as the "most important" factor in full recovery, and certainly in his choice of himself as the "best judge" of whether or not he is fully recovered.

There was great variation in the patients' estimates of length of time required for full recovery. The highest proportion of patients (39%) chose 4–7 weeks. The estimates ranged from as little as one week to more than a year.

In summary, then, in defining full recovery patients used three major criteria: (1) the surgery sequellae must be resolved; (2) it must be possible to resume usual activities; and (3) the physician must corroborate full recovery. Patients are more self-reliant in determining criteria for their full recovery than they are in relation to criteria for hospital discharge.

SOCIOLOGICAL VARIABLES AND RECOVERY DEFINITIONS

The majority of subjects responded similarly concerning recovery. Internal cues—especially strength, feelings, and capabilities—were more important to them than external cues in determining recovery. And most were dependent on the physician in relation to recovery in the hospital, though more self-reliant in relation to this at home. There were, however, a number of striking differences between the several groups. Highlights of these will be presented here. These differences remained in the great majority of instances when the multivariate analysis was carried out.

Socioeconomic Status: The literature supports the notion that socioeconomic status exerts a powerful influence on all types of attitudes and opinions (Kohn, 1969, p. 72). This was found to be so in the results of this study. Its effects were more pervasive than those of any of the other independent variables.

There was a marked inverse relationship between socioeconomic level and percentage of positive responses to recovery factors included in the instrument. Subjects of the upper socioeconomic groups were extremely selective in the choice of factors important to them; they rated comparably few as important recovery cues. The ones chosen showed a great deal of self-reliance. Their own capabilities and independence were most important to them in determining recovery, while cues from others, except the doctor, held little value for them. The lowest socioeconomic group tended to favor physical cues more frequently than other cues in determining their recovery. And, on the whole, this latter group tended to rate the great majority of all factors in the scale as very important in determining recovery.

Ethnic Groups: Black and white subjects tended to view recovery as described in the previous section. Hispanic subjects showed more variation in their views of important recovery factors. They leaned heavily on their feelings and on their families' cues in determining recovery.

Black subjects relied most on their capabilities and physical factors in determining recovery.

White subjects also preferred capability cues most; and external cues were valued little.

Religious Groups: Subjects in all three religious groups preferred capability cues most often in determining their recovery. However, Protestant and Catholic subjects were more responsive to external cues than were Jewish subjects.

Of the three variables thus far presented, the socioeconomic status of the subjects appears to be the predominant influence on responses to the recovery determinants. Through the multivariate analysis it was learned that, for the most part, religious and ethnic group influences were overshadowed by the values of the class of which the subjects were members.

Sex: Female subjects showed a preference for their feelings as recovery determinants, and they were more responsive to the opinions of their families and friends than were male subjects. Men placed greater emphasis on their capabilities, and thus generally estimated shorter recovery periods than did women.

There was a great deal of variation in the responses of subjects grouped according to marital status. They will not be discussed here.

Age: For the majority of age groups studied, age itself did not appear to produce distinctive response patterns. The oldest age group, 61–70 years, was the one exception to this. They showed an obvious tendency toward independence and self-reliance in their responses. They emphasized their own feelings and capabilities strongly in determining their recovery. They regarded external cues from medical and nursing personnel as important less frequently than any other group. They even saw their own opinions of their recovery as more important than the physician's. Self-sufficiency is obviously an extremely important value for patients in this age group, whose independence may be threatened with their advancing years.

Type of Surgery: Patients who had major abdominal surgery and those who had herniorrhaphies tended in most ways to view recovery similarly. The differences found in their responses seemed to be related to the relative extent of the surgery and the recency of the operative day.

Patients who had undergone major abdominal surgery, whether male or female, showed a greater concern for nearly all factors in determining their recovery than did hernia patients. They had apparently experienced more and thus had more from which to recover. This was especially true of factors dealing with feelings. These subjects also showed a greater reliance on the physician's opinion of their recovery than those in the other operative group.

Whether male or female, the major concerns of patients who had herniorrhaphies were centered about their independence and relief of pain. This may be explained by the fact that many of these patients had had their surgery only one or two days prior to the interview and the specific effects of surgery were still very vivid for them.

IMPLICATIONS

The findings of this study have broad implications for health professionals responsible for the care of patients recovering from surgery, most particularly nursing practitioners and nursing educators. Patients determine their recovery from surgery using criteria which they are best fit to judge: their strength, energy, feelings, and perceived ability to resume usual activities and responsibilities. This may be termed a sociological definition of recovery.

In contrast, in their care of patients, health professionals tend to use a medical definition of recovery from surgery, based primarily on wound healing, pain, vital signs, and laboratory data. Decisions about recovery and discharge are made on this basis. The discrepancy between these definitions may account for many difficulties encountered in the recovery period of surgical patients.

The interest that led to this research was occasioned by observation of unexpected delays in patient discharge from the hospital due to new and often minor symptomatology. The reasons for these occurrences were not investigated in this study. However, it may be hypothesized that the patients' criteria for their readiness to leave the hospital may not have been satisfied, and hence the delay. A study of this problem and its financial implications might yield very useful data for designing pertinent nursing care interventions.

With the rising costs of institutional care, third-party payers have imposed stringent rules for the utilization of hospital beds. Currently, discharge criteria are primarily medical in nature. There is little consideration given to social or psychological factors that might influence the patient's readiness for discharge. Delayed discharge and the readmission of patients who were discharged earlier than was appropriate for them have very real financial implications.

The knowledge that patients have their own criteria for readiness to leave the hospital and for full recovery has further implications for nursing practice. If patients are to be truly included in the planning and implementation of their care, their criteria for recovery must be considered. If the overall information gained in this study were formalized into a routine assessment guide for the post-operative patient, many positive outcomes could result.

Post-operative patients could receive the comprehensive care that is so often advocated. Nurses could diagnose and treat patients' responses in the post-operative periods. Needs patients have identified could be met on an individual basis. One source of dissatisfaction the patient-consumer complains of, lack of individualized care, could be removed.

A better mesh of patient and institutional goals could also

be realized. Institutional goals deal with delivering the best care possible, in the shortest possible time, at the least expense, resulting in a satisfied patient. Patient goals are very similar. And, patients are more likely to consider that they have received the best care possible if professionals in the institution understand what the patient's goals are and if these are an integral part of his care.

The findings of this study have implications, too, for nursing education. The information concerning patients' criteria for recovery could and should be included in teaching students at all levels about the needs and responses of the post-operative patient.

The approach used in this study could be a model for students to utilize in the care of any type of patient. Eliciting and responding to the patient's input into his own situation can only improve the care he receives. The several major concerns of patients in defining their recovery have specific implications for nursing intervention. Patients were extremely concerned about their strength and energy levels and their ability to be independent in action and to function post-operatively. Part of this concern may be due to the fact that they were not prepared for the debilitating effects of surgery. The physical and emotional toll of surgery has profound temporary effects on energy levels. Patients should be prepared for these and thus helped to set realistic goals for convalescence. And their attempts at independence should be supported and encouraged.

Another major concern of patients dealt with the emotional impact of the surgical experience. Patients having even the most minor of operative procedures respond emotionally to the threat that surgery imposes. Patients should be prepared for such emotional reactions to surgery and be given the opportunity to ventilate their distress.

Some patients in this study reported that their depression, fear, and crying after the operation frightened them; they wondered if they were "abnormal." Others complained that only their pain was treated—that no one took care of their feelings and "how bad they felt." Attention to all patients' emotional responses to surgery can be a major factor in reducing the trauma and anxiety of the whole experience.

The sociological variables included in this study were found to influence patients' definitions of recovery markedly. In general, the knowledge gained can be used as a guide in the approach to patients from those groups. However, since generalizations cannot be made to all individuals of any group, individual patients' responses should always be elicited and supported in giving care.

Several of these findings may nevertheless serve as overall guidelines in approaching patient care. Patients of the upper socioeconomic group, single persons, and Black subjects emphasized regaining their capabilities after surgery. This should be supported in their care. Patients of the lower socioeconomic groups showed a particular concern for the resolution of the physical consequences of the surgery. This should be recognized and interventions planned to include these concerns.

Female patients, patients having major surgery, and Hispanic patients tended to rely heavily on their feelings and were very responsive to the opinions of their families in determining their recovery. These patients should be given the opportunity to discuss their feelings freely, and family should be included readily, as appropriate, in planning care. Male subjects, who seemed to downplay feelings, should also be given opportunities to ventilate feelings.

Older patients were shown to value their independence post-operatively. This should be recognized and included in care plans.

The major implications of the findings of this study are for the health professionals involved in the care of post-operative patients. Patients have very specific criteria that they use to define their recovery from illness. If these criteria are included in the assessment, planning, implementation, and evaluation of patient care, patient outcomes should be substantially improved.

RECOMMENDATIONS

Recommendations for future study are made in the hope of further developing the construct of recovery. It appears that much more could be learned about the process of recovery if similar studies of the present type could be conducted, but with many modifications.

Cues and categories could be more precisely defined. "Strength and energy" were regarded as primary recovery determinants by patients, as was the "feeling" of recovery. Both were subjectively defined and monitored. More precise definitions could be developed.

This study was concerned with the effects of sociological variables on recovery criteria but not with psychological ones. It is known that personality variables have a pervasive and intrinsic effect on all behavior. A study that included personality factors would greatly increase our knowledge of the recovery construct.

Most patients of the lower socioeconomic status groups rated all factors in the scale as very important. The question arises as to whether the study with its tool as constructed was appropriate in tapping the thoughts and ideas of these subjects. Another study, using methods more suited to the background of these patients, might uncover a more precise definition of recovery for similar subjects.

The patients in this study were specifically selected to determine a baseline definition of recovery. Physically and emotionally, their conditions were essentially uncomplicated. Many of the criteria they used in defining their recovery are probably universal ones. However, to further develop the construct of recovery, studies dealing with patients whose illnesses are very different should be undertaken. The recovery definitions of patients with mental illnesses, chronic debilitating diseases, and life-threatening surgery or illnesses as well as those who have mutilating surgery or illnesses that entail body image and life style changes, would add a great deal to the understanding of this whole construct.

This study was designed to explore recovery definitions from the patient's point of view. However, patients are cared for by a variety of health professionals, most particularly physicians and nurses. It would be very profitable to learn how the definitions of those caring for a group of patients compare with the patients' own definitions. Solutions to some of the problems encountered in the recovery period might be uncovered as a result.

There were wide disparities in patients' estimates of the length of time needed for full recovery. It would be interesting to learn what types of factors influence such estimations. A study made six weeks or more after discharge might answer this question. Such a study could also verify the projections made by patients in this study as to what full recovery really is.

A final recommendation for future study deals with the emotional response of patients to "routine" surgery. This appears to be an extraordinarily distressing part of the surgical experience. It certainly is traumatic for the patient; yet, little is known about it. The topic deserves further inquiry.

This study was conducted in an attempt to determine how patients define recovery. A great deal was learned that can be helpful in better understanding patients' responses during the recovery period. Much that was learned could also be directly applied in the care of patients in the recovery phase of illness. However, very much more is still to be learned about recovery, and it awaits further intensive investigation.

REFERENCES

Burgess, Ann, & Lazare, Aaron. *Psychiatric Nursing in the Hospital and Community.* Englewood Cliffs, N.J.: Prentice-Hall, 1973.

Carlson, Carolyn. "Grief and Mourning." In *Behavioral Concepts and Nursing Intervention.* Coordinated by Carolyn Carlson. Philadelphia: J.B. Lippincott, 1970.

Kohn, Melvin. *Social Class and Conformity.* Homewood, Ill.: Dorsey Press, 1969.

Koos, Earl L. *The Health of Regionville.* New York: Columbia University Press, 1954.

Lindemann, Erich. "Symptomatology and Management of Grief." In *Crisis Intervention.* Edited by Howard J. Parad. New York: Family Service Association of America, 1965.

Mechanic, David. *Medical Sociology: A Selective View.* New York: Free Press, 1968.

Parsons, Talcott. "Definitions of Health and Illness in the Light of American Values and Social Structure." In *Patients, Physicians and Illness.* Edited by E. Gartley Jaco. New York: Free Press, 1972.

Rosenberg, Morris. *The Logic of Survey Analysis.* New York: Basic Books, 1968.

Saunders, Lyle. *Cultural Differences and Medical Care.* New York: Russell Sage Foundation, 1954.

Zborowski, Mark. *People in Pain.* San Francisco: Jossey-Bass, 1969.

Critique

Grace R. Dowling

AS THE authors suggest, if the processes of becoming ill and recovering from illness were better known, nursing assessment could then derive more accurate implications for the care of persons experiencing these processes. Although there is not yet a universal definition of illness, several models have been suggested. Some models are based on a health-illness continuum, while others suggest indicators of levels of wellness or the adequacy of human adaptive processes. The assessment of states of health and/or illness requires collection of data about physical, psychological, and sociological variables. As suggested by the World Health Organization's definition, the concept of health should include more than the absence of illness, and the ability to assess deviation from an optimum state of health is an important nursing skill. Nursing intervention into the process of an individual's becoming ill will have a positive impact on the level of health of the population and on health care costs; nursing care of patients in the process of recovery will be strengthened by knowledge of variables that can facilitate or impede the recovery process.

A sociological definition of illness cites as an indicator of illness the impairment to perform normal role expectations. The research presented in the Kolditz and Naughton study incorporates role expectation as a benchmark for patients who were then asked to rank the importance of other variables in terms of the events of discharge from the hospital and resumption of normal role. The study correctly confines its inquiry to its stated purpose; that is, it attempts to define the relationship between selected sociological variables and the psychological variables represented by patients' definitions of recovery from acute illness in an effort to understand the experience of patients who are recovering from an episode of acute illness, a surgical experience.

The decision to select patients who are recovering from a surgical procedure carries the assumption that the individual was well before surgery, or at least that wellness existed before recognition of the pathological process that required surgical intervention. It should be noted, however, that 33 of the cases were identified as emergency surgery. Whether surgery was scheduled as the result of exacerbation of a pre-existing condition or as a completely new occurrence of illness is not determined, and if the focus of the study were on psychological variables, that determination would be essential. This study, then, represents a first step in developing an understanding of wellness based on patients' interpretations of the level of wellness required for each of two events: discharge from the hospital; and resumption of normal activities—defined as full recovery.

METHODOLOGY

This is a descriptive study of variables related to patients' definitions of recovery. Using appropriate survey research techniques, the authors have related the variables of socioeconomic status, ethnicity, religion, sex, marital status, and age to discharge and full recovery criteria. Information on the relative importance of these variables was obtained and presented in quantified forms in the section on findings of the study.

The study further seeks to describe relationships among the variables and to relate responses to the discharge and full recovery criteria to sociological characteristics of the patients and the type of surgery experienced. Glock (1967, p. xx) has proposed that questions about relations between variables stem from a theoretically grounded expectation as to why the variables ought to be related. He notes that this theory does not include a cause-and-effect relationship, but that variables ought to be related because they are components of a larger entity. As we have seen in this study, specific independent variables, such as sex, ethnicity, age, and religion, were related to the recovery criteria in similar ways as subsets of the overriding category, socioeconomic status. This relationship is not unexpected to those with a knowledge of social conditions in the United States, but the characteristics of the sample should be kept in mind when attempting to generalize from these data. A survey of this type conducted in another cultural setting could provide valuable insight into similarities and differences in sick role behavior in different countries. The study does not attempt to give explanations or to draw inferences. This will be the task of further research building upon the findings presented here. The research does, however, provide a wealth of data on sociocultural background and status related to patient attitudes during the "fifth stage" of illness (Suchman, 1965, p. 114), depicted here as recovery and rehabilitation from a surgical procedure. The findings of the study, therefore, contribute to the growing body of literature on social factors related to responses to illness and medical care.

Parten notes that an optimum sample in a survey should fulfill the requirements of efficiency, representativeness, reliability, and flexibility. The sample should be small enough to avoid unnecessary expense, and large enough to avoid intolerable sample error (Parten 1950, p. 293). Authorities vary in recommending minimum sample size, and they are reluctant to be specific. The researcher, therefore, must consider the alternatives for statistical treatment of the data when determining the minimum number of subjects required for a study.

This sample has met the requirement of efficiency by providing a sample size appropriate to use of the Chi-Square statistic in determining significance. The sample may be said to be representative of the population studied, keeping in mind that clients of medical centers in New York City are most likely to be residents of metropolitan and suburban areas and therefore are not representative of the population of the nation as a whole. Bias was avoided by pre-specifying characteristics of patients in the study to include only patients with uncomplicated herniorrhaphies or other abdominal surgery at a predetermined point in their post-operative period of recovery. No controls were exerted on demographic or other sociological variables, nor was there any assessment of psychological variables. The sample, then, is representative of the population served by the cooperating institutions, except for the exclusion of private patients in all but one hospital. Reliability has been achieved by obtaining cooperation from almost all of the patients who met study criteria in each of the four hospitals on the basis of two visits per week to each institution to collect data. Because no stratification was involved in selection of the sample, flexibility was achieved by permitting the investigators to continue to collect data until they had reached their predetermined sample size of 200 patients.

The procedure followed, with the investigators visiting each hospital twice a week, required nine months to obtain the necessary sample of 200 patients, although the total number of surgical beds in the four institutions was 365. Their fortitude is commendable. The difficult nature of survey research should be taken into account by others who would undertake similar work. Survey research is expensive and time-consuming and requires the physical stamina and willingness to be present when the desired subjects are available. More than physical presence is required, however, when collecting data in a health care setting. Investigators have the additional responsibility of creating attitudes of understanding and cooperation among the staff while at the same time fulfilling their purposes of obtaining the needed data while not interfering with the ongoing care of patients. The vagaries of data collection described in this and other clinical studies should be recalled by others who attempt to do clinical studies without employed research staff. If, as a profession, we believe that clinical studies are essential to developing bases for nursing theory and action, then we must develop the means for adequate support of clinical research.

The technique for data collection was implemented through personal contact by the investigators. An interview schedule was developed to assure consistency in approach, and the questionnaire was reviewed to avoid bias.

The framework of the instrument developed for this study provides a valuable approach to the study of patients' feelings during episodes of illness. The authors derived four categories of concern to patients in developing this instrument. These were physical cues, feeling tone cues, capability cues, and cues from others. These categories can provide a conceptual basis for other clinical studies because they are reality-based and broadly defined. These characteristics will permit others to use this framework with other variables valid in the clinical situation being studied. For example, items within each broad category could be developed around situations of recovery from a life-threatening illness, pre-operative assessment, the postpartum situation, or recovery situations that require substantial modification of the individual's life style. Findings of the present study, in which sociological variables are related to recovery cues, also suggest possibilities for clinical research using experimental designs, as well as for nursing intervention, most obviously in the categories of cues from professional staff and from family and friends.

TREATMENT OF THE DATA

The results of the investigation were presented first as frequencies of responses to items chosen as "very important" on the rating scales. Relationships among the sociological variables and the criteria for recovery that were identified as very important were then tested for significance using the Chi-Square statistic in bivariate and multivariate analyses. In development of the instrument for data collection, the criteria for recovery were derived from patient interviews. In responding to the questionnaire, the patients in the study sample interpreted these criteria without assistance or explanation of terms by the researchers. The findings of the study present, therefore, patients' ratings based on the perceived meaning of each term to the individual, rather than on a set of scientifically derived criteria which could be presented in alternative phrases (for example, by presenting a number of phrases all meaning "return of strength" to assure that the patient's interpretation was consistent).

Although the individual items in the scales are not mutually exclusive, they do fall into the four mutually exclusive broad categories: physical cues, feeling tone cues, capability cues, and cues from others. The cues-from-others category was further subdivided into the categories of cues from professional personnel and cues from family and friends. As noted earlier, the scientific derivation of these categories in this study provides a valuable contribution to nursing research by having developed a conceptual framework for other clinical studies.

The analysis of the data revealed a number of significant relationships indicating that group membership does in fact influence patients' perceptions of readiness for discharge and resumption of normal activities and that socioeconomic status became a very pervasive factor related to perception.

FINDINGS

The authors have carefully identified the limitations of the data. Intervening variables, particularly those of a psychological or emotional nature, were not considered. Further research in this area could employ a similar conceptual framework, and a study could, for example, focus on psychological variables such as prior knowledge, belief systems, or locus of control related to self-assessment of recovery status.

Findings of the study that were not anticipated by the researchers deserve further investigation. Patients' perceptions of an operative experience as a crisis situation should be documented for both major and minor surgical procedures. The post-operative depression noted here could be further studied by use of mood and feeling tone scales, for example as in LaLima's (1976) study of mood during the first 14 days of the post-partum period.

The investigators have identified important areas for further research. They have provided an intense analysis of a group of patients' beliefs about criteria for hospital discharge and full recovery from surgery and have derived a useful framework for studying these beliefs. Further pursuit of the concept of patients' definitions of states of health and illness will not only provide valuable information for nursing practice and nursing education; more knowledge of how individuals define these terms will also be invaluable to those involved in planning for the delivery of health care.

REFERENCES

Glock, Charles Y. *Survey Research in the Social Sciences.* New York: Russell Sage Foundation, 1967.

LaLima, Josephine. "Characteristics of Moods in Primiparous and Multiparous Patients during the First Fourteen Days Post Partum." Ed.D. dissertation, Teachers College, Columbia University, 1976.

Parten, Mildred. *Surveys, Polls, and Samples: Practical Procedures.* New York: Harper & Bros., 1950.

Suchman, Edward A. "Stages of Illness and Medical Care." *Journal of Health and Human Behavior* 6 (Fall 1965): 114–128.

Contributors

Geraldine Allerman, R.N., Ed.D.
Assistant Director of Continuing Education, St. Luke's Hospital Center, New York City

Mary Xenia Wasson Britten, R.N., Ed.D.
Assistant Professor, School of Nursing, State University of New York at Binghamton

Grace R. Dowling, R.N., Ed.D.
Office of Academic Affairs, State University of New York at Binghamton

Doreen Kolditz, R.N., Ed.D.
Assistant Director, Loeb Center, Montefiore Hospital, New York City

Rose Ann Naughton, R.N., Ed.D.
Associate Professor of Nursing, Molloy College, Rockville Centre, N.Y.

Marilyn T. Oberst, R.N., Ed.D.
Director of Nursing Research, Memorial Sloan-Kettering Cancer Center, New York City

Sydney H. Pendleton, R.N., Ed.D.
Associate Professor, School of Nursing, Louisiana State University Medical Center

Sister Aloise Anne Zasowska, R.N., Ed.D.
Dean and Professor, College of Nursing, Niagara University, Niagara University, N.Y.